ESPE – The First 50 Years
A History of the European Society for Paediatric Endocrinology

50

ESPE – The First 50 Years

A History of the European Society for Paediatric Endocrinology

Editor

Wolfgang G. Sippell Kiel

on behalf of the ESPE Council

83 figures, 68 in color, and 16 tables, 2011

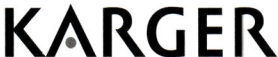

Basel · Freiburg · Paris · London · New York · New Delhi · Bangkok · Beijing · Tokyo · Kuala Lumpur · Singapore · Sydney

Published with the support of

Eli Lilly and Company
Ferring Pharmaceuticals
Ipsen
Merck Serono S.A.
Novo Nordisk Health Care AG
Pfizer Endocrine Care
Sandoz International GmbH

Research and Project Management: Dr. Matthias Georgi, Neumann & Kamp Historische Projekte, Munich, Germany
Members of the project team: Ina Deppe, Katharina Roth, Carola Wagner

Library of Congress Cataloging-in-Publication Data
A catalog record for this book is available from the Library of Congress.

Bibliographic Indices. This publication is listed in bibliographic services.

Illustrations. Every effort has been made to obtain permission for all copyright-protected material. Any omissions are entirely unintentional. The publisher would be pleased to hear from anyone whose rights unwittingly have been infringed.

Disclaimer. The statements, opinions and data contained in this publication are solely those of the individual authors and contributors and not of the publisher and the editor(s). The appearance of advertisements in the book is not a warranty, endorsement, or approval of the products or services advertised or of their effectiveness, quality or safety. The publisher and the editor(s) disclaim responsibility for any injury to persons or property resulting from any ideas, methods, instructions or products referred to in the content or advertisements.

All rights reserved. No part of this publication may be translated into other languages, reproduced or utilized in any form or by any means electronic or mechanical, including photocopy ing, recording, microcopying, or by any information storage and retrieval system, without permission in writing from the publisher.

© Copyright 2011 by S. Karger AG, P.O. Box, CH–4009 Basel (Switzerland)
www.karger.com
Printed in Switzerland on acid-free and non-aging paper (ISO 9706) by Reinhardt Druck, Basel
ISBN 978–3–8055–9868–2
e-ISBN 978–3–8055–9869–9

Contents

IX **Foreword**
Chiarelli, F. (Chieti) and Kelnar, C.J.H. (Edinburgh)

XIII **Preface**
Sippell, W.G. (Kiel)

ESPE History

3 **Beginnings**

13 **Establishment of ESPE (1969–1979)**

23 **Growth and Development (the 1980s)**

34 **Going East – New Members in Central, Eastern and Southern Europe (1990s)**

41 **ESPE Evolves**

50 **Leading World-Wide**

Personal Recollections

63 **ESPE Is in Good Health**
Argente, J. (Spain)

65 **Some Milestones in the Development of Paediatric Endocrinology in Belgium and ESPE**
Bourguignon, J.-P. and Maes, M. (Belgium) on behalf of the Belgian Study Group for Paediatric Endocrinology (BSGPE)

- 71 **We Were Young and Very Enthusiastic**
  Chiumello, G. (Italy)

- 73 **Souvenirs of ESPE : I Remember**
  Czernichow, P. (France)

- 76 **High Scientific Quality**
  Dacou-Voutetakis, C. (Greece)

- 79 **Integration and Globalisation**
  Darendeliler, F. (Turkey)

- 81 **The ESPE Annual Meeting Concerts**
  Drop, S. (The Netherlands)

- 83 **The Future of Paediatric Endocrinology in Spain Is Guaranteed**
  Ferrández Longás, A. (Spain)

- 85 **ESPE Has Been Like a Family**
  Grüters-Kieslich, A. (Germany)

- 88 **Lucky and Privileged to Be a Member**
  Hughes, I. (UK)

- 91 **The Impact of ESPE on Paediatric Endocrinology in Slovenia and Its Surroundings**
  Krzisnik, C. (Slovenia)

- 94 **What ESPE Means to Me**
  Laron, Z. (Israel)

- 96 **A Long Way to ESPE from Behind the 'Iron Curtain'**
  Lebl, J. (Czech Republic)

- 100 **ESPE Turns 50: Many Happy Returns and Best Wishes from Switzerland**
  Mullis, P. (Switzerland)

- 103 **A Greek Adventure**
  New, M. (USA)

- 105 **The Transition of ESPE**
  Rappaport, R. (France)

- 107 **My ESPE: Personal Views and Memories of My Favourite Society**
  Ritzén, M. (Sweden)

- 111 **Fulfilment and Fallibility: The Reflections of an ESPE Secretary (1997–2004)**
  Savage, M. (UK)

- 115 **Happy Birthday to ESPE, a Fine Example of European Integration**
  Sippell, W.G. (Germany)

- 119 **'Back to the Vikings': Paediatric Endocrinology in Denmark**
  Skakkebaek, N.E. and Kastrup, K.W. (Denmark)

- 122 **ESPE from a Personal and Finnish Perspective**
  Voutilainen, R. (Finland)

ESPE Facts

129 Annual ESPE Meetings
129   Overview of the Annual ESPE Meetings
131   Annual ESPE Meetings 1962–2011

192 Secretaries, Treasurers and Honorary Members
192   ESPE Secretaries
192   ESPE Treasurers
192   ESPE Honorary Members

194 ESPE Schools
194   Summer School
197   Winter School

198 Committees and Working Groups
198   ESPE Council Committees and the Chairs in June 2011
198   Other ESPE Committees
199   ESPE Working Groups

200 Consensus Statements

202 Awards and Scholarships
202   Andrea Prader Prize
203   ESPE Research Award
203   ESPE Young Investigator Award
204   Outstanding Clinician Award
205   ESPE Research Fellowship
206   ESPE Clinical Fellowship
209   ESPE Sabbatical Leave Programme
211   ESPE Visiting Scholarship
211   Henning Andersen Prize
213   Travel Grants
213   ESPE-Hormone Research in Paediatrics Prize
214   ESPE President Poster Awards

216 Index to pp. 1–125

Foreword

It is an honour and pleasure for us, the ESPE Secretary General (F.C.) and the President for the 50th ESPE Meeting (C.K.) to contribute a Foreword to this book, which has been commissioned and published to mark this important anniversary for our Society.

We would like to thank Wolfgang Sippell whose idea this was, and who has worked tirelessly to bring the project to fruition in a timely manner. Our thanks also to all Society members who have contributed the reminiscences that follow, and to those whose support has made publication possible, especially Jeff Bolton and Hartmut Wollmann (Pfizer), Anne-Marie Kappelgaard (Novo Nordisk) and Thomas Nold (Karger Publishers).

It is interesting that a Society of the size which ESPE has now become still (as is also clear from many of the following contributions) inspires feelings of being part of a family rather than of an impersonal organisation. Like a family, ESPE has grown dramatically over two generations. We look forward to welcoming around 3,500 delegates to the ESPE 50th Meeting, in contrast to Professor Andrea Prader and the handful of other pioneers at the first meeting in Zurich. Several of the latter are, happily, still with us and present in Glasgow as guests of the Society.

As ESPE has grown in size, it has also developed an increasingly wide range of educational and scientific activities, all of which have been designed, ultimately, to improve care for children and young people with endocrine disorders, not only in Europe but worldwide. The diversity of these activities can be seen by accessing the Society's website (www.eurospe.org), but perhaps we may also be allowed a few personal remarks here.

For one of us (F.C.), the first experience of ESPE was at the Annual Meeting in 1984, organised by Dieter Schönberg in Heidelberg, Since then, as a young paediatric endocrinologist, I was very glad and proud to attend the Annual Meetings (every year) of what I considered, already at that time, the best meetings in Paediatric Endocrinology anywhere in the world. My University colleagues and I aimed to show our best data at ESPE meetings and prepared thoroughly to present and debate our findings.

For many years I dreamt of contributing to ESPE as a Council member. After 2001, when I was elected to Council at the Joint Meeting in Montreal, Martin Savage was a very supportive and kind mentor to me and I learned a lot from his leadership of the Society. In 2003 I was honoured to be elected as Secretary General, initially to serve the Society from 2004 to 2007. In those 3 years, together with Council, I worked hard to modernise the Society, to spread information about ESPE around the world and to attract members from countries outside Europe. This has particularly come to fruition during my second term (2007–2010): approximately 15% of members are now from non-European countries making ESPE one of the most scientifically significant paediatric endocrinology societies worldwide. ESPE Annual Meetings are now very well attended with more than 2,000 delegates coming from more than 90 countries.

I was asked by Council and members to stay one more year as Secretary General until the Glasgow meeting, which marks the 50th Annual Meeting of ESPE, and I accepted with pleasure. I am in no doubt that ESPE has influenced my professional (and personal) life very much, and I will continue to serve our Society in the future, doing my best to help Lars Sävendahl, the new Secretary General, to continue the mission of further improving ESPE activities and scientific meetings.

For the other (C.K.), the first experience of ESPE was at the pioneering 1st joint meeting with the Lawson Wilkins Pediatric Endocrine Society, organised by Pierre Sizonenko in Geneva in 1981, and I have presented data at virtually every meeting since then. I am proud to have served on Council, helped to guide the Society's strategic direction and to be involved with ensuring that our interaction with the pharmaceutical industry continues to reflect the highest ethical standards as these evolve over time. ESPE has always been at the forefront of developing such relationships, which are vital for our scientific and educational activities, in a transparent and appropriate manner.

I have always felt that such activities as the Winter School and, especially, the Clinical Fellowship Programme, which I have chaired for a number of years, go to the heart and soul of what an organisation like ESPE should be about. ESPE has provided educational opportunities for trainee paediatric endocrinologists, initially from Eastern Europe but now including all parts of Europe, Africa, South America, India and China, as ESPE itself has developed to become the premier paediatric endocrine society worldwide.

It is appropriate, I believe, that this 50th Meeting of the Society takes as its theme 'Evidence-Based Paediatric Endocrinology – Its Strengths and Limitations'. This significant milestone in the history of our Society gives us the opportunity to look back at what we know scientifically, to critically appraise the basis of that knowledge and to look to the future as ESPE becomes an increasingly international forum for the exchange of high quality basic scientific and clinical information. We are also continuing the long-standing tradition (as discussed by Sten Drop below) of having a memorable concert during the ESPE evening, given by the Chamber Orchestra of Europe.

For both of us, thinking back over so many Annual Scientific Meetings (and forward to more!), there are, of course, fond memories of particularly outstanding lectures and symposia. We also remember the delight when an eminent senior colleague commented favourably on a poster presented at our first meetings. There has been the continuing pleasure of renewing old acquaintances and making new friends at the Annual Meetings and at other ESPE educational activities, including the Winter and Summer Schools, and elsewhere, discussing collaborative research or clinical matters.

Above all, as we in our turn have become more senior in the Society, we have valued these and other special opportunities to support and encourage our younger colleagues from all around the world, in whose hands the future of paediatric endocrinology, and of ESPE itself, appears to be secure.

Francesco Chiarelli
Professor of Paediatrics and Paediatric Endocrinology,
University Department of Paediatrics, Chieti, Italy
Christopher J.H. Kelnar
Professor of Paediatric Endocrinology,
University of Edinburgh, Edinburgh, UK

Preface

The plan to collect and describe ESPE memorabilia started to evolve in the summer of 1997 when I was sorting and packing the ESPE files into boxes for my successor as Secretary, Martin Savage. Already during my years as Secretary I had realised that the files in the boxes inherited from my predecessors were not as complete as I had expected and that they included almost nothing from ESPE's early days. Fortunately, I soon discovered that ESPE's first Secretary/Treasurer, Henk Visser, had kept his personal, tidy collection of meeting programmes and correspondence from 1962 to 1975 which he readily offered for my use. My own collection started in 1975, so I had continuity, at least in terms of meeting programme booklets. The original intention of presenting a review of ESPE's remarkable development at its 40th anniversary during the Joint meeting in Montreal was neither ideal in terms of the setting nor realistic in view of the workload involved. So we aimed at the 50th annual meeting in Glasgow, the city which had already hosted ESPE's 5th meeting back in 1966.

When looking at the dozens of huge removal boxes packed with paper files at the ESPE secretariat in Bristol, the megabytes of electronic files there and the large collection of historically interesting photos amassed so far, it soon became clear that this project would need professional help to succeed. I found this in Dr. Matthias Georgi, a young historian who, with his team, has specialised in compiling and editing histories on industrial and scientific topics, and I am grateful to ESPE Council for supporting him. Since all relevant paper files, including meeting programmes and photos, have now been scanned, Council and members in the future will have access to a new ESPE Electronic Archive in which every document can be easily searched for and retrieved. This will greatly facilitate Council and committee work, improving continuity since, e.g. previous discussions and decisions on specific topics will be readily available.

The intention of this book was not to describe the history of paediatric endocrinology in Europe – this would require 5–10 times the number of pages – but rather to provide a concise overview of the development of ESPE from a small club of friends to a global scientific society. It should also have a personal touch, so Council selected (in its usual, well-balanced fashion) 21 senior members who enthusiastically volunteered to briefly record their 'Personal Recollections' of ESPE. These are fun to read, and also reflect the charming variety of approaches to this task within Europe. This book should also serve as a reference, compiling the most important facts of all previous ESPE Annual Meetings (a tedious task). This section seems all the more important as none of the many members I have asked have kept all their previous programme booklets, not even most of the former Presidents regarding 'their' ESPE meeting.

I would like to thank all those ESPE members and friends who readily and enthusiastically contributed photos, stories, files and data. Henk Visser, now in his eighties and with an impressive memory, was indispensable for covering the first 15 years; Leo Van den Brande and Ralph Rappaport provided valuable help with details of their terms as Treasurer and Secretary. All former ESPE Presidents whom I was able to approach promptly helped to fill in most missing details. This general cooperation and overall support from the membership demonstrated that the old ESPE spirit of friendship still lives on. I am very grateful to Matthias Georgi and his team for their expert support, in particular to Ina Deppe, Katharina Roth and Carola Wagner of 'historische-projekte.de', to Joanna Voerste, my former ESPE secretarial assistant for her excellent job of translating texts and polishing up my English drafts, and to Thomas Nold at S. Karger Publishers: without them this ESPE history project would not have become a reality.

Wolfgang G. Sippell
Professor (emeritus) of Paediatrics and Paediatric Endocrinology
Christian-Albrechts-Universität zu Kiel, Kiel, Germany

ESPE History

ESPE History

Sippell WG (ed): ESPE – The First 50 Years. A History of the European Society for Paediatric Endocrinology.
Basel, Karger, 2011, pp 3–12

Beginnings

A Club Is Founded: ESPE's Prenatal Period (1962–1964)

In 1962, Professor Andrea Prader, Director of the University Children's Hospital (Kinderspital) in Zurich, invited 26 paediatricians and endocrinologists who had attended the 4th Acta Endocrinologica Congress in Geneva from July 3rd to July 7th and were interested in foetal and paediatric issues to attend an informal post-conference meeting in Zurich. The idea was to discuss specific problems and questions concerning paediatric endocrinology in a smaller group, which would allow a greater in-depth exchange of ideas and experience. The catalyst for Prader's invitation was his disappointment with the programme of the Acta Endocrinologica Congress, which had not included any paediatric endocrinology. Andrea Prader wrote about this later in a brief history of the ESPE: 'I knew from personal experience that the few participating paediatricians would learn much in general endocrinology but would not have an opportunity to discuss their specific problems. [...] The meeting brought together for the first time the few and mostly young European investigators in the new speciality and proved to be very stimulating and fruitful for all of us.'[1]

Thirty-two paediatricians and endocrinologists attended the meeting (see illustration, p. 4). There were no British colleagues because none had attended the Acta Congress in Geneva. The participants were lodged in a hostel near the Kinderspital, some of them sharing a double room. The first meeting of the European paediatric endocrinologists opened on the evening of Sunday 8th July 1962 with a reception at the Hotel Sonnenberg, Zurich. The scientific meeting started next morning with a session on the anterior pituitary. Nine topics were dealt with during the meeting, which ended on Tuesday evening with a boat trip and dinner. The conference was a great success, and it was agreed that the participants of this unofficial 'Paediatric Endocrinology Club' should meet once a year, always in a different European country.

---

1 Prader A: History of the ESPE. Horm Res 1989;31(suppl 1). See also for the development of Paediatric Endocrinology as a discipline Fisher DA, Laron Z: The early history of pediatric endocrinology. Pediatr Endocrinol Rev 2003;(suppl 1):66–91 + Erratum: Pediatr Endocrinol Rev 2003;1:127.

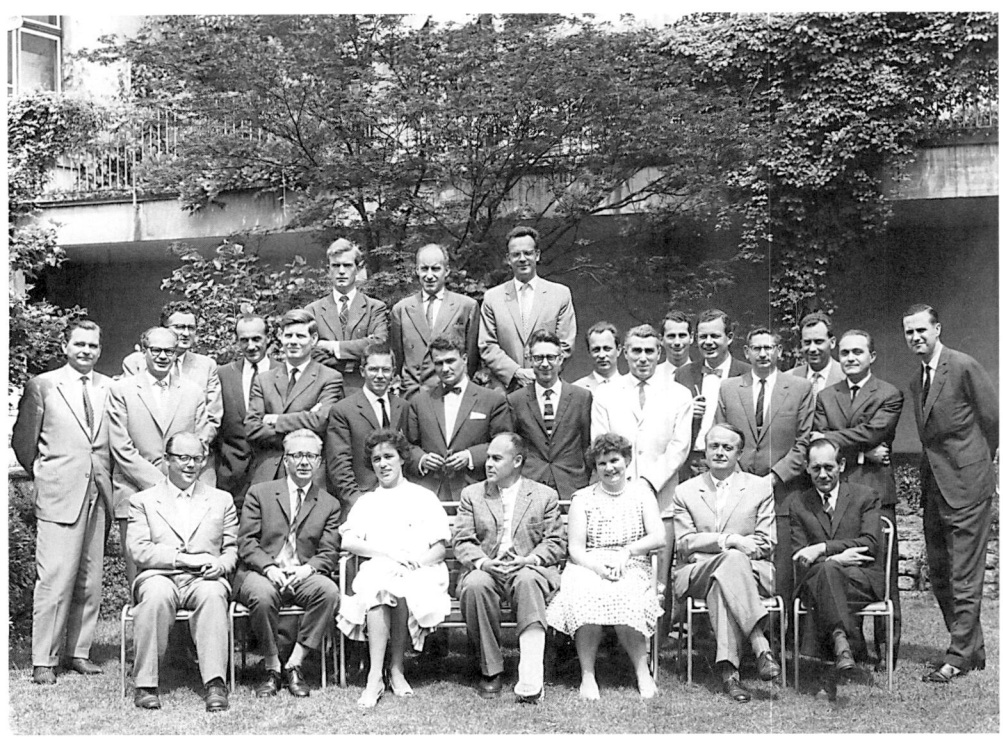

The Founding Meeting of the 'Paediatric Endocrinology Club' in Zürich in July, 1962. From left to right, front row: Henning Andersen (Denmark); Andrea Prader (Switzerland); Ruth Illig (Switzerland), Hans Habich (Switzerland); Gertrud Mürset (Switzerland); Alfred Schwenk (Germany); Carl-Gustav Bergstrand (Sweden). Second row: Egon Werner (Germany); Robert Steendijk (The Netherlands); Henk Visser (The Netherlands); Pierre Ferrier (Switzerland); Jacob Van der Werff ten Bosch (The Netherlands); Lucien Corbeel (Belgium); René François (France); Markus Vest (Switzerland); Dieter Knorr (Germany); André Spahr (Switzerland); Andreas Fanconi (Switzerland); Jürgen Bierich (Germany); Zvi Laron (Israel); Karl Schärer (Switzerland); F.J. Huix (The Netherlands); José M. Francés Antonin (Spain). Third row: Lars R. Nilsson (Sweden); Gerhard Stalder (Switzerland); Emile Gautier (Switzerland).

The second meeting was organised in 1963 in Groningen by Hendrick (Henk) Visser who was later to become the first Secretary/Treasurer of ESPE, a position which he held until 1971. It was attended by 31 participants, predominantly paediatric endocrinologists, from nine different European countries (see illustration, p. 5), as well as 20 Dutch guests. Several British colleagues also took part, including Sir Douglas Hubble (Birmingham), the doyen of European paediatric endocrinologists and editor of the first European textbook of paediatric endocrinology which was published in 1969.[2]

Henk Visser was successful in attracting three sponsors from the industry to support the meeting financially. An extensive social programme was also included:

2   Hubble D: Paediatric Endocrinology. Oxford, Blackwell Scientific, 1969.

DEPARTMENT OF PAEDIATRICS
STATE UNIVERSITY
59 OOSTERSINGEL
GRONINGEN
THE NETHERLANDS

GRONINGEN,

SECOND MEETING "PEDIATRIC ENDOCRINOLOGY CLUB" GRONINGEN, THE NETHERLANDS

MAY 5th - MAY 8th 1963

- Dr. Walter Swoboda
- Dr. (Mrs.) Jacqueline de Mayer-Cuignard
- Dr. Henning J. Andersen
- Dr. Jean Bertrand
- Dr. René François
- Dr. Michel Pierson
- Dr. Raphael Rappaport
- Dr. Douglas Hubble
- Dr. Noel Raine
- Dr. Methven Cathro
- Dr. Jürgen Bierich
- Dr. Gustav A. von Harnack
- Dr. E. Werner
- Dr. Walter Teller
- Dr. A. Schwenk
- Dr. Zvi Laron
- Dr. J.H.P. Jonxis
- Dr. Koos van der Werff ten Bosch
- Dr. Hendrick K.A. Visser
- Dr. José M. Francés Antonin
- Dr. Carl G. Bergstrand
- Dr. Lars R. Nilsson
- Dr. A. Prader
- Dr. Ruth Illig
- Dr. Gertrud Mürset
- Dr. Pierre Ferrier
- Dr. Markus Vest
- Dr. Emile Gautier
- Dr. Heskel M. Haddad
- Dr. Thomas Hill Shepard

Dr. Rob Steendijk

List of participants of the second meeting in Groningen, 1963 with their signatures.

activities were organised for the 'ladies' and the third day of the conference was devoted entirely to an excursion to the Dutch tulip fields.[3]

The scientific programme was spread over 2 days. In his opening address, Henk Visser reported that so many papers had been submitted in advance that some of them had had to be rejected. He advocated the establishment of a society with clearly defined membership criteria and with meetings open to all those who were interested. A committee should decide which papers were to be accepted. His idea was to establish a European society which would give new impulses to paediatric endocrinologists throughout Europe.[4] Cooperation with endocrinologists in other scientific associations, and particularly in the American Society for Pediatric Research (SPR), which had been in existence since 1929, would open up further opportunities.

Indeed, in the years after World War II many of the participants had been in the USA as Fellows at the Johns Hopkins Hospital, Baltimore, Md., either under Dr. Lawson Wilkins, the founder of paediatric endocrinology, or one of his many disciples (the 'Wilkins boys'), and had taken their first enthusiastic steps in this new subspecialty there. Wilkins himself had attended the 6th International Congress of Paediatrics, which was held in Zurich in 1950 under the presidency of Professor Guido Fanconi, and had presented there his revolutionary new life-saving cortisone treatment for congenital adrenal hyperplasia (CAH). He told Andrea Prader, then a resident at the Kinderspital, everything he knew about CAH, and Prader visited Wilkins in Baltimore in the summer of 1951. This was the beginning of the highly successful collaboration between Europe and America in the new field of paediatric endocrinology.[5]

At the 1964 Business Meeting in Hamburg agreement was reached on a more effective organisation of the Club, the first Council was elected and Henk Visser was appointed as first Secretary/Treasurer. He presented a draft constitution for the Society which was to be voted on at the meeting the following year. The name of the newly established association was to be the 'European Society for Paediatric Endocrinology'. There should be a maximum of 30 Founding Members 'with an active scientific interest in paediatric endocrinology', who, ideally, had attended all previous meetings. Council unanimously agreed on a list of 30 Founding Members who should be invited to attend the next meeting (see box on p. 7), which was to be the official Founding Meeting of the ESPE.[6] Henk Visser wrote to the proposed Founding Members in February 1965 and asked for their approval. They also received a draft

---

3   Programme of the second meeting of the Paediatric Endocrinology Club, Groningen, 1963.
4   ESPE archives, speech from H. Visser at the second meeting of the Paediatric Endocrinology Club, Groningen, 1963.
5   Fanconi A: Zum Hinschied von Prof. Dr. Andrea Prader. Paediatrica 2001;12:50–52; Fisher DA: A short history of pediatric endocrinology in North America. Pediatr Res 2004;55:716–726.
6   ESPE archives, letter from H. Visser: From the Secretary to the proposed Founding Members, Groningen, 1st February, 1965.

The Founding Members of the ESPE

Austria
Walter Swoboda

Belgium
Paul Malvaux

Denmark
Henning Andersen

France
Jean Bertrand, René François, Michel Pierson, Raphaël Rappaport, Pierre Royer

Germany
Jürgen Bierich, Dietrich Knorr, Walter Teller, Alfred Schwenk, Egon Werner

Great Britain
Methven Cathro, William Hamilton, Douglas Hubble, James M. Tanner

Israel
Zvi Laron

The Netherlands
Robert Steendijk, Koos van der Werff ten Bosch, Henk K. A. Visser

Spain
José M. Francés Antonin

Sweden
Carl-Gustav Bergstrand, Lars R. Nilsson

Switzerland
Emile Gautier, Andreas Fanconi Jr., Ruth Illig, Gertrud Mürset, Andrea Prader, Markus Vest

of the constitution, which had been translated from Dutch to English by William Hamilton, Glasgow.[7]

The ESPE Is Born (1965–1968)

The ESPE was officially founded at the meeting in Copenhagen in 1965. In the first ESPE constitution, which was adopted on August 10, 1965, the aim of the Society was stated as follows:

'The Society shall promote knowledge of Paediatric Endocrinology in the widest sense. [...] The Society shall organize Annual Scientific Meetings for personal communications and conferences on subjects of general interest. The Society shall further research in Paediatric Endocrinology by bringing together people with an active interest in Paediatric Endocrinology, by arranging exchange visits of members and their collaborators, by promoting joint projects and by other means desired by the Society. The Society shall also stimulate contacts with other Societies with like aims.'[8]

---

7   ESPE archives, letter from H. Visser to W. Sippell, Rotterdam, 16th February, 2002.
8   Constitution and Regulation of the European Society for Paediatric Endocrinology (accepted at the 4th Annual Meeting, Copenhagen, 10th August, 1965).

Constitution and Basic Organisation

With the conversion of the Club into a society, commonly agreed, formally regulated structures and processes for scientific discussion, decision making and publications were established.

The constitution stipulated the conditions of membership. The scope of the different committees and important responsibilities within ESPE were regulated. The Business Meeting served as central advisory and decision-making body for the membership which, according to the wording of the constitution, was also known as the Annual General Meeting. Here the members discussed where and when the next Annual Meetings would be held and where the abstracts were to be published, and decisions were made about accepting new members. The election of Council Members and voting on amendments to the constitution were also tasks for the Business Meeting.

Council was responsible for managing ESPE – Article 4 of the constitution stated 'the Society shall be governed by a Council'.[9] It normally consisted of six members, the first being Andrea Prader, Henk Visser, Henning Andersen, Jürgen Bierich, René François and William Hamilton.[10]

New Council Members could be proposed either by Council or by any Ordinary Member. A rotation system was in operation whereby two Council Members retired each year. Council Members were elected to serve for a period of 3 years, with the possibility of standing again for a further term. During ESPE's first decades the annually convened Council Meeting was traditionally held on the evening before the start of the Annual Scientific Meeting, thus enabling final preparations for the Business Meeting.

The Secretary played a major role, chairing both the Council Meeting and the Business Meeting. He was appointed from among the Council Members and dealt with all important matters regarding the Society and Council. In particular, he fostered a regular exchange of information within ESPE and was responsible for preparing the minutes of the various meetings. The Secretary also represented the ESPE in Europe and overseas.

The Society's finances were also regulated in the constitution: it was agreed that from 1966 a yearly membership fee of USD 10 would be charged. This also fell within the Secretary's sphere of responsibility since, until the constitution was changed in 1972, he also acted as Treasurer. In fact these duties turned out to be more arduous than originally expected: by mid-1966 only 12 members had paid their dues to the Treasurer, Henk Visser![11]

---

9 Constitution, p 1.
10 ESPE archives, letter from H. Visser, 30th January 1964.
11 ESPE archives, letter from H. Visser: To all members, from the Secretary, 2nd November, 1966.

Becoming an ESPE Member

The ESPE constitution foresaw different categories of membership. In addition to Ordinary Members it was possible to admit so-called Corresponding and Honorary Members. All candidates for membership were expected to play an active scientific role in the field of paediatric endocrinology and to support the ESPE as an organisation. In addition, narrower geographical criteria applied for Ordinary Members than for Corresponding and Honorary Members: they had to come from a European country. Membership status affected voting rights. Corresponding and Honorary Members were allowed to play an active part in the Business Meeting, but were not permitted to vote. They could be proposed by Council and were elected at the Annual Meeting.

How could a paediatric endocrinologist apply for full membership? During the early years it was common for Ordinary Members to invite a guest, whom they later put forward as a candidate for full membership, to attend the Annual Meeting. In accordance with the constitution, the proposed new Ordinary Members were presented to the Business Meeting for election. Applicants had previously submitted their CV and list of publications to Council and, following a brief introduction by the sponsoring Ordinary Member, were permitted to make a brief presentation, as laid down in Article 6.[12]

Scientific Programme and Scientific Communication

The Annual Meeting was at the centre of ESPE activities and committees. This was the forum for discussing important research results and exchanging ideas. A fundamental aspect during ESPE's early years was the organisation and further development of the scientific programme, the main objective of which was described as the 'presentation and discussion of new original studies'.[13] Short presentations were made at the first Club meetings; at the very first meeting in 1962, 10 presentations had been made, each followed by a detailed discussion in which all participants enthusiastically joined. The different speakers had been invited by Andrea Prader and covered questions concerning steroid purification from urine by paper chromatography, the use of anabolic steroids in dwarfism and the metabolic effects of human growth hormone.[14]

The framework of the Annual Meeting was regulated by the constitution. It was to be divided into different scientific sessions, each session should consist of seven to

---

12 ESPE archives, letter from H. Visser: To all members, from the Secretary, 25th July, 1966; constitution, p 1.
13 Constitution, p 2.
14 ESPE archives, summaries Annual Meetings; Programme of the first meeting of the Paediatric Endocrinology Club 1962, Zürich.

eight presentations, each to be followed by a discussion.[15] In 1966, the scientific programme comprised four sessions with a total of 33 presentations.[16]

The concept of scientific quality assurance was an important aspect from the beginning: The speakers were encouraged to submit abstracts of their talks before the conference to allow a pre-selection. According to the statutes, the President and Secretary were responsible for programme planning.[17]

Gradually the preparation and presentation of the scientific programme became more polished and professional. At the 5th ESPE Annual Meeting in 1966, where 20 ESPE members and 50 guests gathered at the Royal Hospital for Sick Children in Glasgow, each scientific session was introduced by a chairman who had experience in the subject matter in question.[18] At the 6th Annual Meeting, which was held in Haifa in 1967, there were five scientific sessions. The first session on perinatal endocrinology was chaired by Andrea Prader. It opened with the first invited lectures (30 min) at an ESPE meeting, presented by Claude and Dorothy Villee from Harvard Medical School, who talked on steroid hormone synthesis in the foeto-placental unit. In the following sessions under the chairmanship of Michel Pierson, Henk Visser and Douglas Hubble the conference participants considered the thyroid, steroids, and adipose tissue and obesity. The subject of the fifth session, which was chaired by Jürgen Bierich, was the pituitary.[19]

The number and form of presentations grew with the increasing specialisation within the sub-speciality of paediatric endocrinology. In Haifa, for example, a distinction was made between sessions with Invited lectures which lasted from 20 to 30 min and sessions in which short papers, which lasted 10 min and were followed by five minutes for discussion, were presented.[20]

In a letter to all members, Henk Visser described the Haifa-meeting as 'a great success in every respect'. He praised the quality of the scientific programme and indicated that this year the abstracts had been sent to all the members prior to the meeting: 'The scientific programme was very good and all of you received the abstracts from Zvi Laron.'[21] 80 participants, 21 of whom were ESPE members, had attended the meeting.[22]

Regular routines and channels of communication evolved within ESPE. The Secretary's Newsletter to the members and the releases reporting on planning progress for the Annual Meeting issued several times a year by the President, were important, as was the receipt of a meeting programme with details of both the scientific events and the social programme. A list of expected conference participants and of

---

15 Constitution, p 2.
16 ESPE archives, summaries Annual Meetings.
17 Constitution, p 2.
18 Agenda for Annual General Meeting, 6th September, 1966.
19 Programme Annual ESPE Meeting 1967, Haifa.
20 Programme Annual ESPE Meeting 1967, Haifa.
21 ESPE archives, letter from H. Visser: From the Secretary to all members, 1st October, 1967.
22 ESPE archives, summaries Annual Meetings.

all sponsoring firms and institutions was dispatched prior to the conference. A lively exchange of letters between the Secretary and the different Presidents bore witness to the cooperative, warm and friendly tone which was frequently a feature of this correspondence.

The ESPE provided its members and the conference participants with a platform for publishing the research results which had been presented at the meetings. In 1964, 33 abstracts from the previous Annual Meeting were published in *Acta Endocrinologica*, and in 1965 35 abstracts were printed in the same journal.[23] According to the constitution, one of the duties of the President and Secretary was to 'arrange for publication of the communications or abstracts of these'.[24] Soon after the founding of ESPE agreement was reached on binding specifications for editing papers and abstracts in preparation for publication. Following discussion at the Business Meeting in Glasgow in 1966, President Hamilton introduced a new system of instructions which was accepted by the members.[25] Henk Visser explained the underlying motivation in a letter to the members in December 1966 as follows: 'Members accepted a proposal by Council to prepare abstracts according to instructions from President and Secretary, to maintain highest possible standards.'[26]

In the early years ESPE cooperated with different journals. After initially having also negotiated with *Helvetica Paediatrica Acta* and the *Israel Medical Journal*, abstracts were published from 1967 to 1973 in *Acta Paediatrica Scandinavica*. 1974 saw the start of cooperation with the international, primarily USA-based journal *Pediatric Research*.[27] From 1968 on, the abstracts were also printed every year in bound form in the ESPE meeting programme booklet.

The Personality of the New Society

The move towards a formal membership with eligibility based on objective criteria, and the development of regulated organisational routines and decision-making processes meant it was possible to combine different objectives. The young subspecialty of paediatric endocrinology could evolve at a high standard in research-oriented discussions in a small circle of experienced and ambitious experts. The endeavour to establish and improve scientific standards is evidenced by the concrete impulses and

23 ESPE archives, summaries Annual Meetings.
24 Constitution, p 2.
25 Agenda for Annual General Meeting, 6th September 1966; ESPE archives, letter from H. Visser: From the Secretary, to all members, 2nd December, 1966.
26 Agenda for Annual General Meeting, 6th September 1966; ESPE archives, cf. to this issue: letter from W. Hamilton: European Society for Paediatric Endocrinology. Publications of Papers read at the Fifth Annual Meeting Glasgow, September 1966, undated.
27 ESPE archives, letter from H. Visser: From the Secretary to the Council Members, 20th June, 1967; ESPE archives, summaries Annual Meetings; ESPE archives, letter from H. Visser: From the Secretary to all members. Short notes of the 9th Annual General Meeting at Lyon, 12th March 1971; Short notes Annual ESPE Meeting, 1971.

innovations emanating from the Annual Meetings. The main focus was on a concentrated scientific exchange of the latest research results and on safe-guarding scientific quality, thus ensuring the integrity of the findings. The Annual Meeting also meant that the research results would be disseminated to a specialist audience. Structures were created under the ESPE umbrella which enabled and encouraged scientific communication. One very important aspect was the platform ESPE provided for publications. Discussions and publications increased awareness of new knowledge and insights, enabling them to be taken up, criticised and further developed.

In the medium and long term, it was possible to create structures for scientific communication which were effective well beyond the confines of the meeting and to specifically promote research in paediatric endocrinology. In the late 1970s and early 1980s, it became clear just how important the efforts and work of the ESPE pioneers really was.

All members were very well known to each other, which explains how Council was able to deal discreetly with an uncomfortable and largely unknown episode in ESPE's history: Because of his affiliation to a national socialist organisation during the Third Reich, one of the ESPE Founding Members was not granted an Israeli visa to attend the sixth Annual Meeting, which was being held in Haifa/Israel with Dr. Zvi Laron as President in 1967. Council and the President were faced with the question as to how they should deal with this issue. They decided to confront the member with this allegation in a personal discussion. He assured them that his membership in the national socialist organisation had been unavoidable in view of his position at the time as a doctor in the public healthcare service, that he had never been involved in working in the concentration camps or similar activities, and had never participated in any anti-Jewish activities. ESPE Council trusted the personal assurances of their fellow colleague.[28]

During the years to 1971, in which the Annual Meetings were held in Glasgow, Haifa, Vienna, Malmö, Lyon and Zurich, the number of ESPE members increased to 60. In addition, there were nine Corresponding Members (mainly from the USA) and one Honorary Member.[29] The meetings were organised entirely by the respective President and his co-workers as 'Local Organising Committee'.

---

28 ESPE archives, letter of H. Visser to W. Sippell, 15th November, 2010.
29 Cf. ESPE membership development in this book, p. 191.

Establishment of ESPE (1969–1979)

Cooperation and New Impulses

In the late 1960s, the ESPE strove to combine research efforts in the fields of paediatrics and endocrinology. In 1968 Walter Swoboda organised the 7th ESPE Annual Meeting in Vienna in cooperation with the European Club for Paediatric Research.[30] In the programme preface the two Secretaries, Henk Visser and Ettore Rossi, outlined their motivation:

'This is the 10th meeting of the European Club for Paediatric Research and the 7th meeting of the European Society for Paediatric Endocrinology. In an attempt to concentrate the congress activities of paediatric research workers it was proposed at our last meetings to try a combined meeting of those two groups. We hope confidently that this attempt will prove to be successful and agreeable!'[31]

The meeting, which was held in the Neues Institutsgebäude of Vienna University, went very well. In September, Henk Visser wrote to Walter Swoboda: 'Dear Walter, the meeting was a great success in every respect. Scientifically the program was the best we had so far for both societies. Socially the program was also excellent.'[32]

The number of registrations received in the spring of 1968 had led Swoboda to expect 300 participants; in the end there were 159, of whom 77 were guests and 44 accompanying persons.[33] At this meeting Corresponding and Honorary Members were elected for the first time. Andrea Prader had proposed Maria New, Edna Sobel, Lytt Gardner and Judson Van Wyk, all from the USA, as Corresponding Members and Sir Douglas Hubble (Birmingham, England) as the first Honorary Member.[34]

---

30 ESPE archives, letter from H. Visser to all members, 1st October 1967.
31 Programme Annual ESPE Meeting 1968, Vienna.
32 ESPE archives, letter from H. Visser to W. Swoboda, 5th September, 1968.
33 Laron Z: Combined Annual Meeting of the European Society for Paediatric Endocrinology and the European Club for Paediatric Research. Israel J Med Sci 1969;5:131.
34 ESPE archives, letter from H. Visser to the Council Members, 5th August 1968.

The 8th Annual Meeting was held in Malmö in June 1969, shortly before the 7th Acta Endocrinologica Congress in Stockholm.[35] New ideas for organising scientific cooperation within ESPE were discussed. In Vienna the members had suggested giving a more informal character to the discussions and presentations held during the Annual Meetings and Carl-Gustav Bergstrand, the President in 1969, wanted to follow up this idea. In a letter to the members regarding the forthcoming conference he wrote: 'The scientific programme has not been definitely arranged but there will be at least two full sessions reserved for free papers. Main topics are still under discussion and the members who have any suggestions are welcome to write me.'[36]

New aspects arose during the course of the meeting. One subject was the financing of research: Henk Visser had already started negotiations with the pharmaceutical industry on financing a research fellowship, and he also suggested running various laboratory workshops in the future.

This was put into action as early as the 9th Annual Meeting in Lyon in 1970: on the third day the conference moved to the Pasteur Institute, where two round tables on laboratory techniques were held. The subjects dealt with were androgen determination and competitive binding techniques. Preparation of the scientific programme was more broadly distributed so that the main responsibility no longer rested with the President alone, who, from 1970, was supported by an Organising Committee.

The 10th ESPE Annual Meeting, in Zurich in 1971, was brought forward to the 8th to 12th of May in order to fit in with two other conferences: from the 5th to 7th of May the Second International Symposium on Growth Hormone was being held in Milan, followed by the Annual Meeting of the Swiss Paediatric Society from the 14th to 16th of May. The Presidents of the ESPE anniversary conference were José M. Francés and Andrea Prader, and Professor Guido Fanconi was appointed as Honorary President. José Francés/Barcelona had set up the endocrine clinic at the Kinderspital in Zurich, together with Andrea Prader, during his time as a resident there; he died unexpectedly a few months after the 10th Annual Meeting.[37] The members of the Organising Committee that year were Andrea Prader, Ruth Illig, Gertrud Mürset and Milo Zachmann.[38] One hundred and forty participants attended the meeting. As the subject of growth hormone had already been covered comprehensively at the meeting in Milan, other topics were chosen for the ESPE meeting: congenital adrenal hyperplasia, testosterone and testes, male pseudohermaphroditism, normal and precocious puberty, and the hypothalamus-pituitary-

---

35 ESPE archives, letter from C.G. Bergstrand to the members: Information No. 1, 1969; ESPE archives, letter from C.G. Bergstrand to the members and guests: Information No. 2, 1969; Programme Annual ESPE Meeting 1969, Malmö.
36 ESPE archives, letter from C.G. Bergstrand to the members: Information No. 1, 1969.
37 G. Knorr-Mürset, pers. commun., 27th April 2011.
38 ESPE archives, letter from A. Prader, R. Illig, G. Mürset, M. Zachmann, November, 1970.

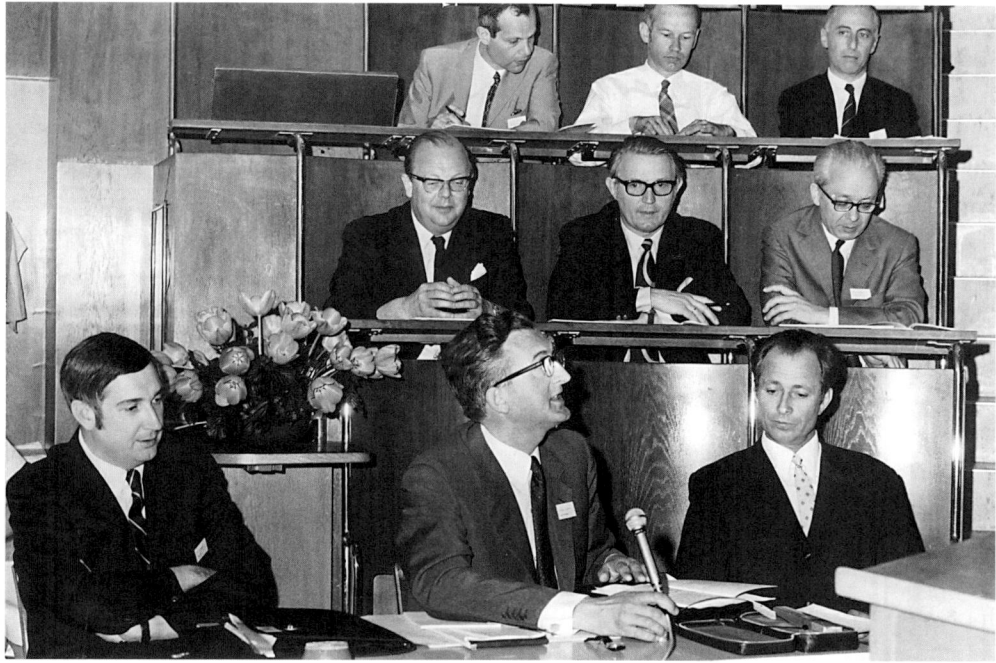

Henk Visser speaking at the 10th Anniversary ESPE Meeting 1971 in Zurich. From left to right, front row: Milo Zachmann; Henk Visser; Dieter Knorr. Second row: Henning Andersen; Walter Swoboda; Andrea Prader. Third row, far right: Jean-Claude Job.

thyroid axis.[39] This year there was particular emphasis on psycho-endocrinological questions. The American psychologist, John Money, spoke on the subject of 'Development of Sexual Identification and Optimal Timing of Surgical Correction of Ambiguous Genitalia'. Group discussions and workshops on psycho-endocrinology, congenital adrenal hyperplasia and steroid methodology took up the third day of the conference (see above illustration).[40]

1971 saw some important changes when Henk Visser and William Hamilton retired from the Council. Visser also resigned as Secretary and Treasurer, and was succeeded as Secretary by Milo Zachmann and as Treasurer by Leo Van den Brande.[41]

The members approved several changes to the constitution during the 11th Annual Meeting in Louvain in 1972. The new Secretary had made several suggestions in advance of the meeting, giving members the opportunity to bring in their own thoughts and ideas.[42] Separation of the offices of Secretary and Treasurer was fixed in the constitution. A further change concerned the Annual Meeting. Article 4

39   ESPE archives, letter from A. Prader to H. Visser, 11th November 1970.
40   Programme Annual ESPE Meeting 1971, Zürich.
41   Programme Annual ESPE Meeting 1971, Zürich.
42   ESPE archives, letter from M. Zachmann, 15th May 1972.

was changed to read 'the President shall hold office for one year and shall organize, in collaboration with the Secretary, the Treasurer and Council, the Annual Scientific Meeting of the Society'. In Article 7 the establishment of an Organising Committee, which was to be appointed each year by the President and Council, was anchored in the constitution. The Committee was responsible for planning the programme, choosing the speakers and should 'arrange for the publication of the communications or abstracts.'[43] A further change was made to the constitution in Paris in 1974: the annual membership fee should no longer be fixed at USD 10, but agreed on year by year.[44]

The Society Expands

The ESPE membership doubled during the 1970s. In 1971 there were 60 members, in 1972 there were 70, and 97 in 1976. By 1979, the number of ESPE members had increased to 127, while in the same period the number of Corresponding Members increased from 9 to 16. There was still just one Honorary Member.[45]

The number of participants at the Annual Meetings was also increasing, so that soon there was talk about 'problems of increasing members and the increasing difficulties in organising Annual Meetings'.[46] Organisation of the Annual Meeting was changing to cope with the larger number of participants. From 1972 (Louvain) on, because of the increasing numbers of abstracts and in order to keep within the time limit, parallel sessions covering very different topics were organised; it was no longer possible for one person to attend all talks or join in all discussions.[47] Because of the large number of participants at the Combined ESPE/ESPR Meeting in 1976 in Rotterdam, scientific posters were exhibited and discussed informally during the lunch break for the first time. Guided poster tours were introduced in 1984 in Heidelberg to counteract the opinion that posters were second class scientific presentations. An expert on the topic in question led a group of interested colleagues from poster to poster, asking the author to present the study and its results in a few minutes and to answer questions from the audience. This oral presentation and discussion was particularly helpful for those investigators who came from non-English speaking countries. Organisation of guided poster tours is very

---

43 Constitution and regulation of the European Society for Paediatric Endocrinology (accepted at the 4th Annual Meeting, Copenhagen, August 10th, 1965, and revised at the 11th Annual Meeting, Louvain, 8th September, 1972).

44 Constitution and regulation (accepted at the 4th Annual Meeting, Copenhagen, August 10th, 1965, and revised at the 11th Annual Meeting, Louvain, September 8th, 1972, and the 13th Annual Meeting, Paris, September 13th, 1974).

45 ESPE archives, list of members, 1971; ESPE archives, list of members, 1972; ESPE archives, list of members, 1976; ESPE archives, list of members, 1979.

46 Minutes of Council Meeting, 30th and 31st January 1976, Rotterdam.

47 Programme Annual ESPE Meeting 1973, Bergen; Programme Annual ESPE Meeting 1974, Paris.

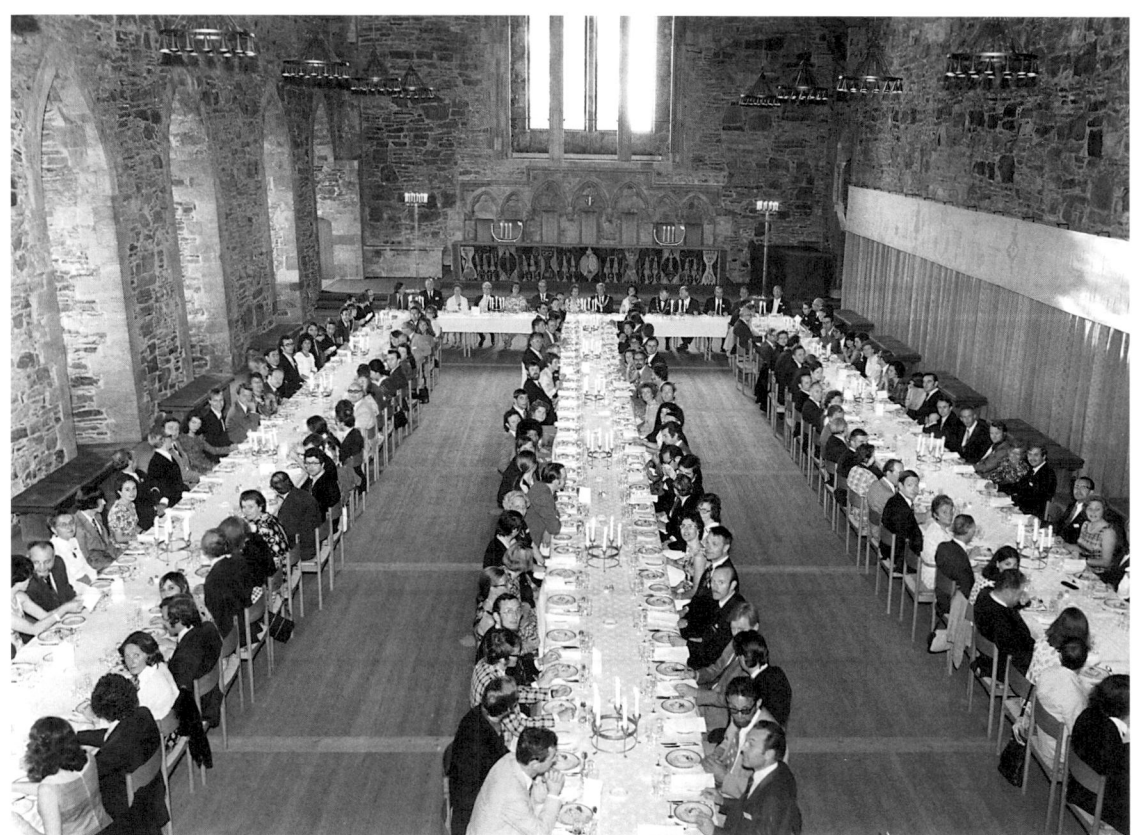

Annual Dinner at Håkonshallen during the 12th Annual Meeting in Bergen, 1973.

work-intensive, and it is sad that they are no longer generally part of every ESPE meeting nowadays.

The growing interest in the Annual Meetings and in ESPE was seen on the one hand as a success, but on the other hand, from the mid-1970s, it gave rise to heated discussions. Leading members expressed fears that ESPE's high scientific standards were being endangered. The system of parallel sessions (since 1972), the growing number of free papers submitted and the large number of new members were criticised. In a letter to Milo Zachmann, Pierre Sizonenko expressed concern 'that many new members have been elected and I am not quite sure that they all fulfil the requirements and aims of the Society. Some of them are not really involved in endocrine research work. This consequently brings to the Society a submission of papers which are not compatible with the quality required and therefore when accepted, lead to unnecessary parallel sessions.'[48]

48   ESPE archives, letter from P. Sizonenko to M. Zachmann, 7th November 1975.

He recommended the introduction of poster sessions – a suggestion which was implemented in the following year.[49]

The 15th Annual Meeting of the ESPE was held in 1976 as a Joint Meeting with the European Society for Paediatric Research. There were seven larger plenary sessions and two poster sessions in addition to 21 scientific sessions.[50] A different emphasis was also placed on content: Council felt 'that more attention should be given to basic science in future meetings, notably when selecting invited speakers, since for many active paediatric endocrinologists it is difficult to keep their knowledge concerning basic (molecular, biochemical) endocrinology up to date'.[51]

Council considered the quality of the scientific contributions. In 1976 'Selection of abstracts and the improvement of quality of papers' was discussed as Item 1 on the agenda.[52]

In view of the numerous suggestions for candidates for membership, the Council Members took their task of pre-selection very seriously. In 1975, three of the nine persons who had been proposed to the Secretary for membership were considered unsuitable – 'either because some council members feel the scientific requirements are not fulfilled, or because the candidates have not yet presented a paper at an Annual Meeting'.[53] They also resolved 'to apply more strict criteria for admission of members in the future'.[54] In 1977, the Council considered only 10 of the 17 candidates proposed to the Secretary to be suitable.[55]

There were ideas of linking participation at the Annual Meetings to age ('seniority') and membership fees. A suggestion to this effect from a leading member did not meet with the Council's approval, but 'led to a more general discussion of the Society's future'.[56]

The Council Members agreed that stricter regimentation would not be helpful, 'but would only reduce the scientific quality of the meetings and make the Society into a "club of old friends"'. It was therefore decided to 'have a liberal policy for the invitation of guests at Annual Meetings' – this should apply especially for young research workers and scientists from countries where there were only a few ESPE members. The old rule, whereby every member could bring only one guest to the Annual Meeting, should not be applied too strictly. ESPE was particularly keen to open its Annual Meetings to scientists from east European countries; to this end Henk Visser should use the communication channels afforded by the European

---

49 Minutes of Council Meeting, 30th–31st January, 1976, Rotterdam.
50 Programme Annual ESPE Meeting 1976, Rotterdam.
51 Minutes of Council Meeting, 14th January 1977, London.
52 Minutes of Council Meeting, 30th–31st January 1976, Rotterdam; ESPE archives, letter from M. Zachmann, 8th May, 1976.
53 Minutes of Council Meeting, 24th September 1975, Berlin.
54 Minutes of Council Meeting, 24th September 1975, Berlin..
55 Minutes of Council Meeting, 14th September 1977, Cambridge.
56 Minutes of Council Meeting, 14th September 1977, Cambridge.

Society for Paediatric Research to make the meeting better known there. At the same time Council confirmed that 'by contrast, the rules for membership admission should continue to be at least as strict as up to now, and selection of new members should be mainly based on scientific merit and not on 'diplomatic' or 'political' reasons.'[57]

New tasks and challenges gave rise to lively debate within ESPE as the highly dedicated scientists were faced with questions and problems which affected the decisions to be made regarding the future and goals of the Society. In spite of the strict entry and selection criteria, ESPE's democratic structure permitted and promoted internal change. This strong foundation enabled ESPE to take on important new tasks from the mid 1970s.

European Training Programme and First International Studies

From 1976 on, at Leo Van den Brande's suggestion, the idea of a Europe-wide training programme had been widely discussed.[58] His vision was to start with a course lasting four to six weeks.[59] Henk Visser wrote to Wolfgang Sippell in 2002: 'In 1976 Leo Van den Brande was the first to start the discussion on paediatric endocrinology training in Europe. This was the beginning of a very successful teaching programme of ESPE, which goes on until today'.[60]

In 1977, Ralph Rappaport was elected as Secretary and Pierre Sizonenko was elected as new Treasurer. Ten new members were admitted in this year.[61]

At the end of the 1970s, the ESPE addressed new scientific tasks. The Society cooperated with the European Thyroid Association in evaluating a neonatal screening programme for hypothyroidism which the ETA had just carried out with the support of many ESPE members.[62]

At the ESPE Annual Meeting in Ulm in 1979, where Walter Teller was President, a stricter ruling regarding payment of membership fees was agreed as a reaction to the increasing financial constraints. Article 2 of the constitution now stipulated that: 'Membership will expire for any member who has not paid the annual fee for three years'.[63]

---

57 Minutes of Council Meeting, 14th September 1977, Cambridge.
58 Minutes of Council Meeting, 30th–31st May 1976, Rotterdam; cf. first suggestion of Leo Van den Brande at the Business Meeting in the previous year: Minutes of Annual Business Meeting, 1975.
59 Minutes of Council Meeting, 30th–31st May 1976, Rotterdam.
60 ESPE archives, letter from H. Visser to W. Sippell, 16th February 2002.
61 Minutes of Annual Business Meeting, 1977.
62 Minutes of Annual Business Meeting, 1978.
63 Constitution and Regulation, revised at the 18th Annual Meeting, 20th June, 1979, Ulm; Minutes of Annual Business Meeting, 1979.

Joint Meetings with the LWPES

The idea of opening the Annual Meetings for American colleagues and of holding Joint Meetings with the North American Lawson Wilkins Pediatric Endocrine Society (LWPES) had been discussed in correspondence between Henk Visser and Milo Zachmann as early as 1972. In a letter dated November of that year, Visser enthusiastically reported:

'Dear Milo, I have just returned from a short trip to the United States. I visited Johns Hopkins and had a long discussion with Claude Migeon. [. . .] I think our Society and the American Society should interchange as much as possible. The secretaries should send each other the programs of meetings and at the next meeting in Bergen I propose to discuss the possibility to open our meeting for members of the American Society. The American group apparently plans to organise workshops on paediatric endocrinology [. . .] I think it would be a good idea to organise these conferences as a joint enterprise of both Societies.'[64]

Zachmann welcomed Visser's approach; however, he pointed to some reservations from within ESPE. Some members feared 'that our meetings would be swamped with Americans, while no one or only a few could attend the meetings in the States from the European side'.[65] In 1976, Council welcomed the idea of a Joint Meeting on condition that it was held in Europe,[66] whereupon Pierre Sizonenko started negotiations with the LWPES for a Joint Meeting to be held in Geneva in 1981.[67] In 1980, it was agreed that 'there will be combined selection of the abstracts with the American Group [. . .] to achieve an adequate balance between Europe and the US for oral presentations and posters'.[68] The Joint Meeting was considered to be a great success by both sides and it was agreed to hold another Joint Meeting in 4–5 years.[69] At the suggestion of the LWPES[70] the second Joint Meeting was held in 1985 in Baltimore. The organisers were Salvatore Raiti and Claude J. Migeon. Jerusalem was chosen as the venue for the third Joint Meeting in 1989: This was the start of close cooperation and intense professional exchange which has endured to the present day.

---

64 ESPE archives, letter from H. Visser to M. Zachmann, 28th November 1972.
65 ESPE archives, letter from M. Zachmann to H. Visser, 5th December 1972.
66 Minutes of Council Meeting, 30th–31st May 1976, Rotterdam.
67 Minutes of Annual Business Meeting, 1977.
68 Minutes of Annual Business Meeting, 1980.
69 Minutes of Annual Business Meeting, 1981.
70 Minutes of Council Meeting, 26th March 1982, Geneva.

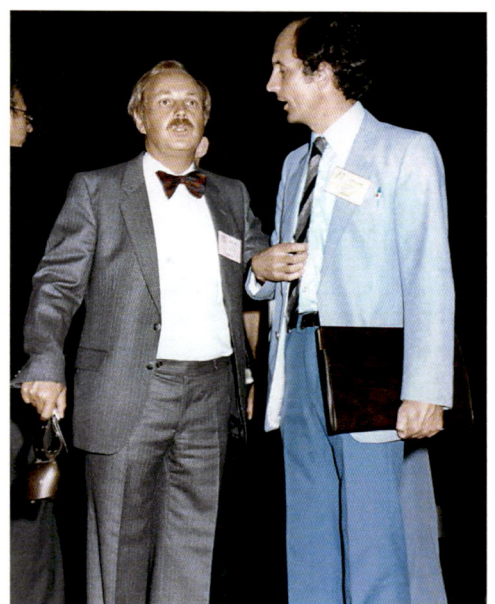

Pierre Sizonenko with Ieuan Hughes holding the gathering bell (an original Swiss cowbell) as symbol of the Joint Meetings at the first Joint Meeting with LWPES in Geneva, 1981.

Love, ESPEcially

'When you join a society, there are always three categories of people', says Trudi Knorr, and places her hand on her husband's arm. 'There are the ones that you dislike immediately, there are the ones that you like immediately and there are the ones that leave you indifferent. Dieter to me was the second category, but nothing more.'

Dieter Knorr and Trudi Mürset, 2 of the 30 Founding Members of ESPE, first met at the very beginning of 'their' Society: at the informal meeting of European paediatricians with an interest in endocrinology in Zurich in 1962. Both of them – 'but separately!' – enthusiastically became part of the small ESPE 'family'.

In 1975, a tragic mountain accident changed both of their lives. Dieter Knorr lost his wife and the mother of their five children.

In the time that followed this sad incident his relationship to Trudi Mürset slowly began to change. Eventually she left her home and her work with Andrea Prader in Zurich and moved to Munich to face a completely new challenge: taking care of a family with five teenagers. 'I felt this could be my path', she recollects. And also: 'in the beginning this new job was more demanding than a busy day in the endocrine clinic at the Kinderspital'.

At the time, the whole Society shared the gradually evolving love of Dieter and Trudi, and one Israeli colleague put it in a nutshell: 'At least that is one positive thing that ESPE has accomplished!'

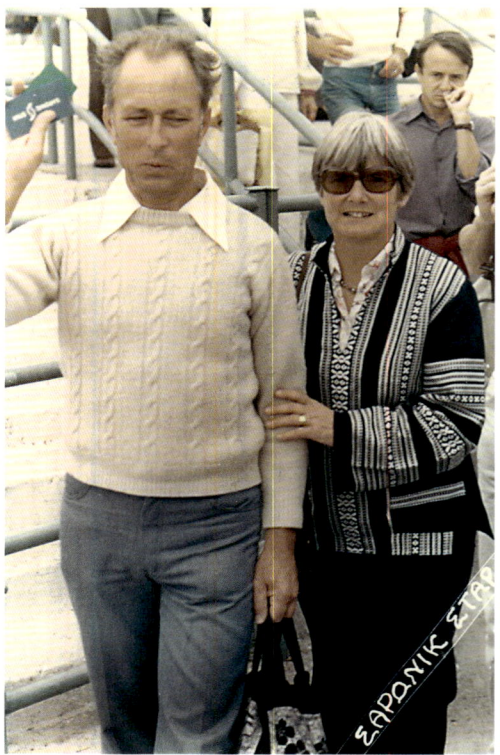

Dieter Knorr and Trudi Knorr-Mürset, Annual Meeting in Athens, 1978.

ESPE History

Sippell WG (ed): ESPE – The First 50 Years. A History of the European Society for Paediatric Endocrinology.
Basel, Karger, 2011, pp 23–33

Growth and Development (the 1980s)

The Society and the Pharmaceutical Industry

Following the phase in the 1970s, in which ESPE established itself as a scientific organisation and laid down the basic rules for the Society, in the 1980s it developed into that institution which is recognised world-wide today as a leader in the field of paediatric endocrinology. The focus of ESPE's work and the topics discussed in Council changed. In addition to the Annual Meeting, a growing number of programmes, fellowships and prizes enabled ESPE to expand its scientific network and, in particular, to support and promote younger researchers.

These 'ESPE products', as Paul Czernichow refers to them in his recollections, were made possible by the generous support afforded to the Society by the pharmaceutical industry. In the mid-1980s money from the industry began to flow more freely into research and to the ESPE. The principle reason for this was the development of recombinant molecular genetic technology and the biosynthesis of human growth hormone, one the first hormones to be produced in this way, theoretically in unlimited amounts. This opened up very lucrative perspectives for industry compared with the very limited, expensive and complex extraction of the hormone from the pituitary glands of corpses, which had been the only method of producing the hormone until then. Cooperation with endocrinological societies such as the ESPE was now more interesting for the pharmaceutical industry, while the endocrinologists also recognised a new source of financial support and, in turn, approached the companies with ideas and suggestions.

This collaboration was advantageous for both parties. However, it soon became clear that hard and fast rules must be agreed on to avoid developments which might result in ESPE being influenced by the industry. One problem was that the companies which supported ESPE wanted to be adequately represented, particularly at the Annual Meetings. This was a problem for the first time at the Annual Meeting in Zurich in 1986. The main sponsor ignored the ESPE membership rule, whereby every member was entitled to bring one guest, and brought several busloads of (uninvited) paediatricians to the meeting. The crush was so great that many members could not get into the auditorium. They were appalled by the way in which access to *their* meeting had been manipulated.

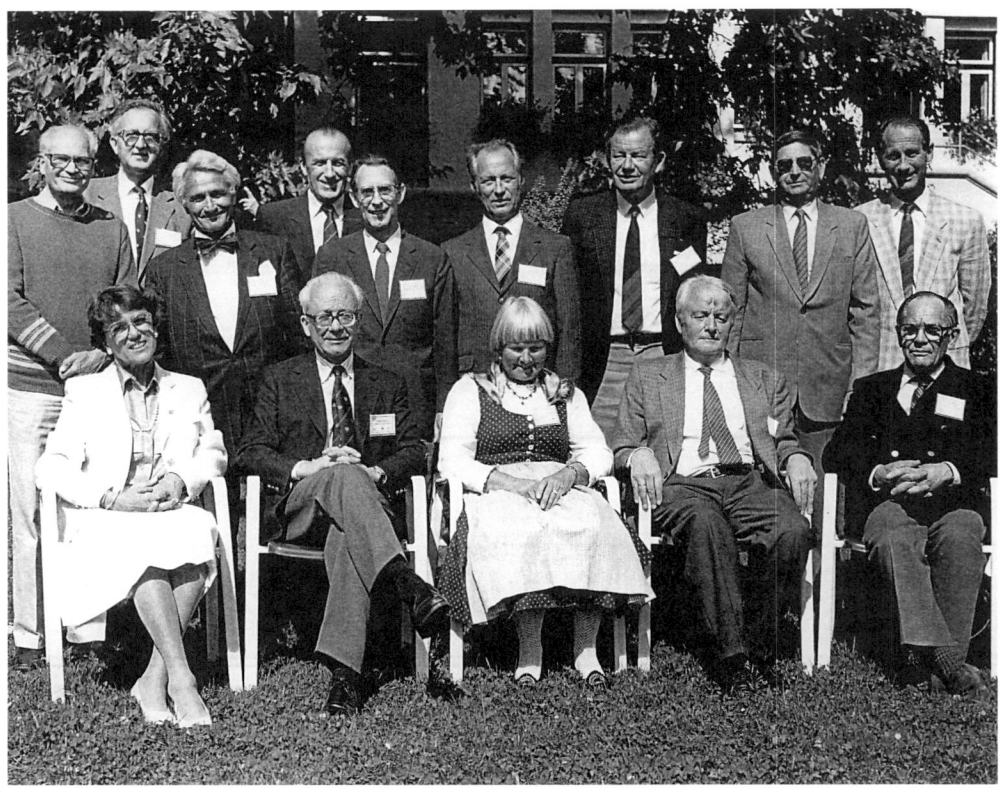

Group picture of the 1962 meeting attendants at the 25th Annual Meeting in Zürich 1986. From left to right, front row: Ruth Illig; Andrea Prader; Gertrud Knorr-Mürset; Alfred Schwenk; Carl-Gustav Bergstrand. Second row: Robert Steendijk; Henk Visser; René François; Pierre Ferrier; Markus Vest; Dieter Knorr; Jürgen Bierich; Zvi Laron; Andreas Fanconi.

A further serious problem was the pressure which was being exerted on ESPE by different sources to recommend a particular product or company, or to support the activities of a single firm.[71]

During preparations for the next meeting in Toulouse in 1987, Council decided that 'the Society would not allow any particular company to dominate the social or business proceedings at the Annual Meeting through undue involvement in any particular event.' In addition, the then Secretary, Al Aynsley-Green, was asked to make detailed suggestions on how to reduce the pharmaceutical industry's influence.[72] He wrote to the companies, impressing on them that the ESPE must remain completely independent. The Society would not permit the sponsoring of Satellite meetings during a scientific conference, or allow firms to use the meeting programme to advertise their own meetings. The rule allowing every member to invite only one guest was to be

71 Minutes of Annual Business Meeting, 1987.
72 Minutes of Council Meeting, 22th–23th May 1987, Toulouse.

strictly adhered to, although the Secretary and President would be permitted to invite additional 'guests of merit'. Donations from companies would no longer be dedicated to individual events, but would go into a single account to finance the meeting.

The pharmaceutical industry and ESPE were never in disagreement; the focus was always on the joint promotion of paediatric endocrinology and ESPE, while at the same time allowing no doubt to be cast on the scientific independence of the Society.

ESPE Summer School

In 1983, several members expressed the wish for a teaching programme targeted especially at young investigators. On November 25th 1985, an extraordinary meeting between the Secretary, Al Aynsley-Green, the Treasurer, Michel Aubert, and Paul Czernichow was held in Paris to discuss a teaching programme.[73] Paul Czernichow reported that the pharmaceutical company Ferring had offered to support such a project with SEK 150,000 each year for the next 5 years. This would be a no-strings-attached donation. With the 25th anniversary of ESPE coming up in 1986, Paul Czernichow felt it was important to reach a decision quickly and thus demonstrate the importance ESPE attached to the promotion of junior colleagues. In the light of the ongoing discussion in ESPE about the influence of industry, it was considered particularly important that all responsibility for the development and control of this programme should remain with ESPE. The Society would be responsible for the organisation, the selection of candidates, for inviting the speakers and evaluating the courses.[74]

In view of the size of the donation, it was considered reasonable that Ferring should be the only sponsor. This sponsorship would be acknowledged by allowing the company to distribute advertising material (e.g. in a conference bag) during the conference and to display an advertisement. The donation would cover the expense of accommodation for all participants and speakers during the course, which would run for up to two and a half days. In order to save money it was decided to run the new course in conjunction with the Annual Meeting. Another advantage in this was that many participants and speakers would be there anyway, and there was usually enough time to fit the Summer School round the meeting so that it would not conflict with other commitments.

At a Council Meeting in January 1986, the name 'ESPE Summer School' was agreed on for the teaching programme, and a diversity of backgrounds should be considered as a positive factor when selecting participants. During the following months possible topics to be dealt with at the Summer School were discussed. Since time was too short to organise a Summer School for 1986, the first one was held at Chateau de Bonas near Toulouse in 1987. 22 participants were selected from 44 applications. Paul Czernichow was appointed as first chairman of the selection committee, the Summer

---

73 ESPE archives, Minutes of Extraordinary Meeting, 25th November 1985, Paris.
74 ESPE archives, Council Discusssions 17–18th January 1986, Geneva.

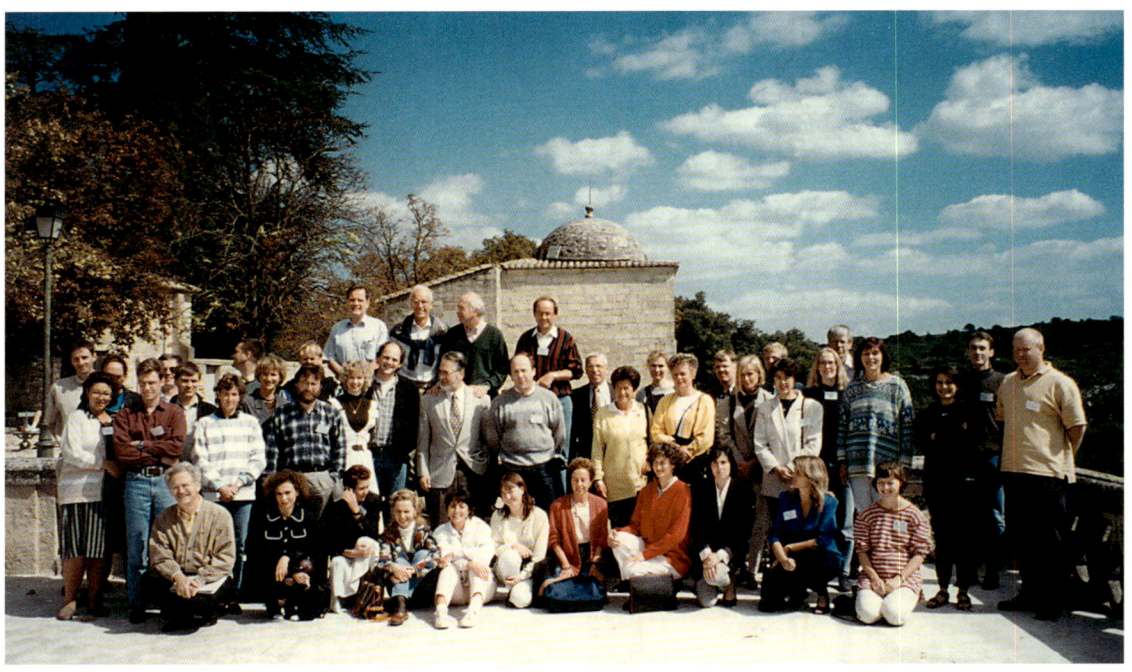

The participants of the ESPE Summer School in Uzés near Montpellier, 1996.

School Steering Committee. First of all it was necessary to establish the selection criteria for participants, and the fundamental decision was taken that the Summer School should not simply be an introduction to paediatric endocrinology. 'It was decided that the ideal participant should be between 30 and 35 years old, that they should have a good background in general paediatrics, and that the candidate should have formally decided to become a paediatric endocrinologist'.[75]

The course should cover the scientific basics of paediatric endocrinology, clinical application and the discussion of case presentations. A limited number of topics should be covered in detail rather than attempting to impart an understanding of all aspects of paediatric endocrinology in two and a half days. The subjects dealt with at the first Summer School were growth and growth factors, perinatal growth and energy expenditure, and intersex (figure in 'Personal Recollections' by Czernichow, p. 74).

Over the years, the ESPE Summer School has flourished and provided a unique opportunity for training in paediatric endocrinology. It has also fostered personal interrelationships between the future ESPE members within the ever-growing Society, resulting in collaborative research projects and publications from former Summer

---

75 ESPE archives, Minutes of Council and co-opted advisors for the Summer School 1987, 13th–14th January 1987, Paris.

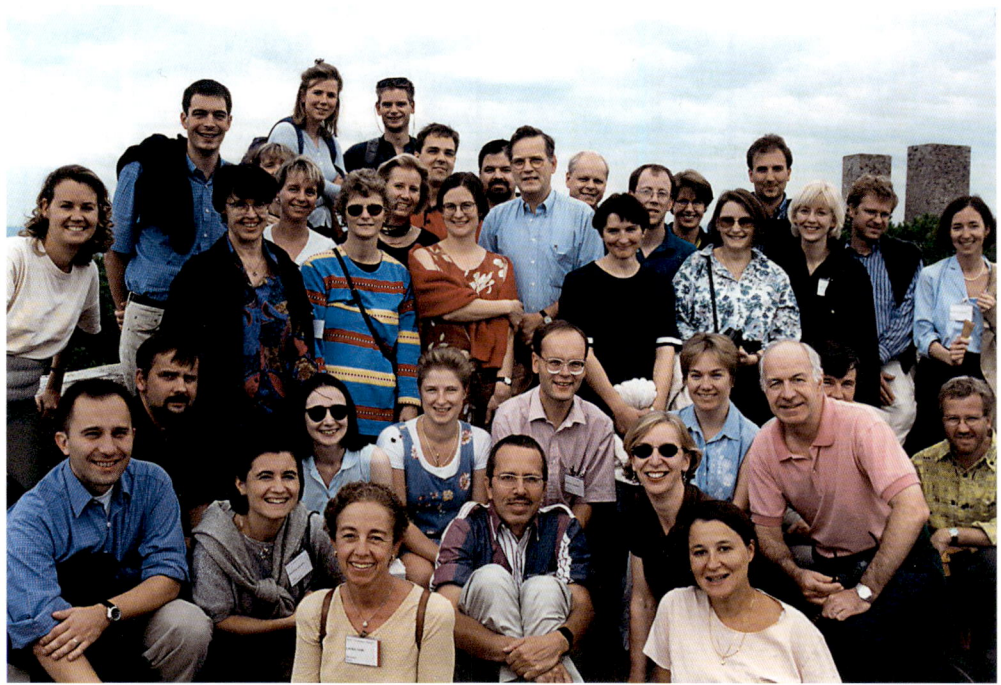

Enthusiasm among the participants of the ESPE Summer School in Warsaw, 1999.

School students. Interest in the ESPE Summer School continues to increase and today many applicants come from outside Europe.

Prizes and Fellowships

Henning Andersen Prize

At the Annual Business Meeting in 1985, Al Aynsley-Green presented 'a major new initiative from the Society relating to a means to improve the quality of abstract submission and to encourage research groups through the formation of an annual ESPE prize for the best abstract submitted to the Annual Meeting'.[76] The group whose abstract scored the highest number of points in blind ranking received SFR 2,000, and the author who presented the paper received a medal. This paper would also be presented first in a Plenary session. The award was named the Henning Andersen Prize after the deceased founding member 'who was one of the fathers of ESPE and of paediatric endocrinology in Europe',[77] and was awarded for the first time in 1986 to Marc Maes.

76 Minutes of Annual Business Meeting, 1985.
77 Minutes of Annual Business Meeting, 1985.

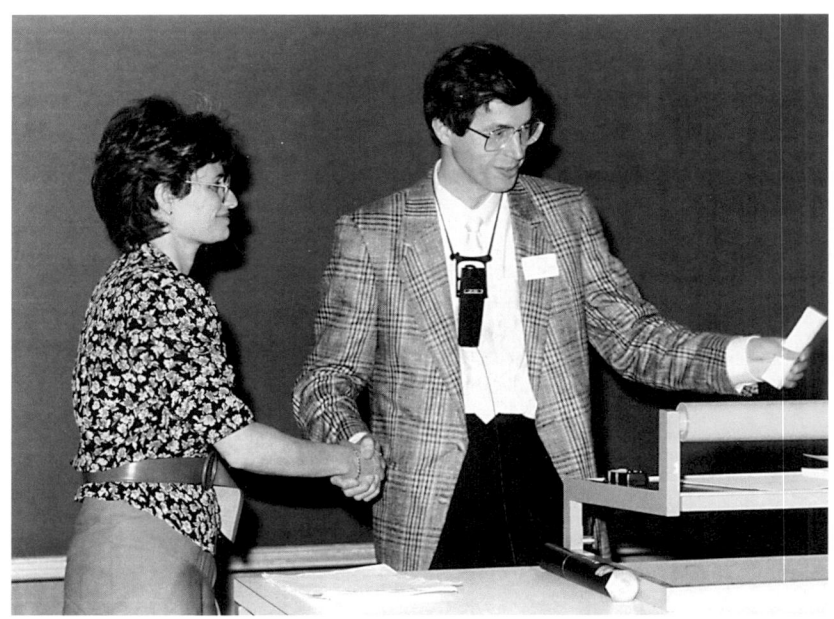

Gila Maor, winner of the Henning Andersen Prize at the Annual Meeting in Copenhagen 1988, with Niels Skakkebaek, ESPE President, 1988.

Andrea Prader Prize

In 1987, the Swedish company, KabiVitrum, agreed to make a substantial sum of money available each year for a prize which would be awarded annually. This was to be presented to young researchers below the age of 40 who were working in the field of growth. Council asked to be allowed to extend the circle of recipients and to establish the prize as ESPE's highest award. The prize, worth SEK 35,000, should be awarded without age restriction to a still active member who had influenced the development of paediatric endocrinology and made a decisive contribution in this area. This accolade was conferred for the first time on the recently retired ESPE founding father, Professor Andrea Prader, who 'kindly agreed to his name being applied to this award'.[78] Candidates should be proposed by the members. The Selection Committee consisted of the ESPE Secretary, Kabi's medical director and three respected senior ESPE members. The first Andrea Prader Prize was awarded in 1988 to Milo Zachmann at the Annual meeting in Copenhagen.

---

78 Minutes of Annual Business Meeting, 1987.

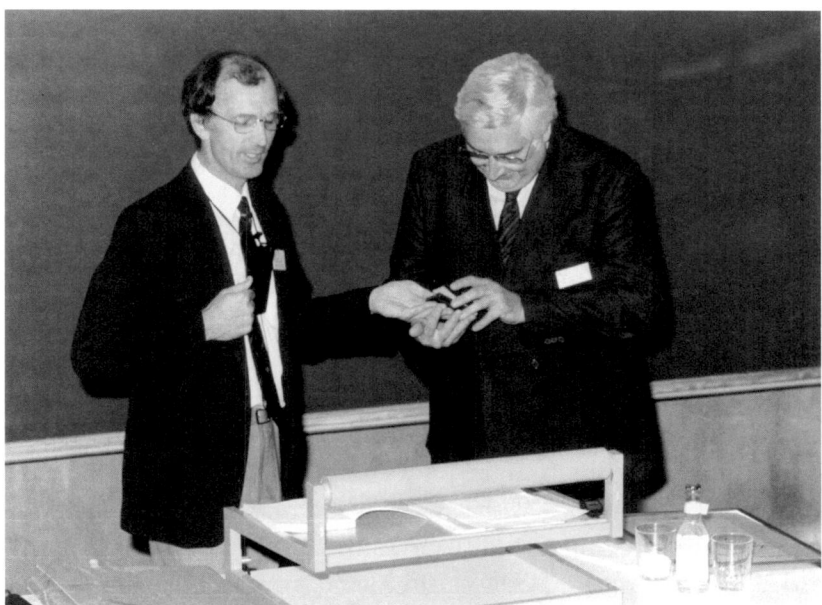

Milo Zachmann receiving the first Andrea Prader Prize from ESPE Secretary Ieuan Hughes at the Annual Meeting in Copenhagen, 1988.

ESPE Research Fellowship

In 1989, the then Secretary, Ieuan Hughes, proposed that the ESPE should introduce a Research Fellowship as successor to the Nordisk Grant for the Study of Growth, which had been instigated in 1978 by Henning Andersen, Andrea Prader and Henry Brennum, the then director of Nordisk Insulinlaboratorium Gentofte/Copenhagen, to enable young paediatric endocrinologists to learn and carry out research in a respected laboratory. The applicant and the host laboratory should submit a joint project application and applicants (age limit of 35) should come from ESPE countries.[79] In 1990, the successor, Novo Nordisk generously agreed to finance several ESPE Research Fellowships, starting with USD 100,000 in the first year, increasing to USD 180,000 in the second year. These cover two to three long-term Fellowships which run for 2 years, and three to four short-term Fellowships of 3–6 months' duration.[80]

Ethical and Medical Questions

The abstracts and their quality had occupied the ESPE since the 1960s. When selecting the abstracts for the Annual Meeting, the members of ESPE Council were concerned

---

79 Minutes of Annual Business Meeting, 1989.
80 Notes from the Meeting to establish ESPE Research Fellowships, Copenhagen, 14th November 1990.

that ethical standards were not being observed in some cases. There were three specific problems: in some abstracts there was no indication that informed consent to take part in a study had been obtained from the parents and the child. Other abstracts reported the repeated taking of blood samples from healthy children, although this offered no benefit to the children themselves. Other studies were submitted in which invasive tests which did not directly benefit the patient had been performed on sick children. At the Annual Business Meeting in 1986, it was recorded 'that the ethical dilemmas would remain within the confidential discussion of the Council, but that this was an aspect which required further open discussion'.[81] On the abstract form in 1987, it was stated for the first time that 'Council will have the right to reject any abstract that presents studies with dubious ethical conditions'.[82] The discussion continued, and from 1990 all submitted abstracts had to show evidence that the author had obtained approval for the study from the local ethical committee. This measure clearly reduced the number of abstracts with a questionable ethical background.

In 1984, on the initiative of Jean-Claude Job, ESPE tackled problems in medical practice, in particular the potential abuse of growth hormone, by setting up a Working Group on the Use of Human Growth Hormone. Its goals were to define the current situation regarding the prescribing of HGH, to improve diagnostic criteria in the broad field of hypopituitarism, and to develop opportunities for conducting joint studies.

Growth hormone therapy was soon to be the cause of great disquiet in the paediatric endocrinology fraternity, although neither ethical problems nor abuse were the reason.

A Deadly Disease due to Contaminated Batches of Extractive Human Growth Hormone

Undoubtedly the most painful episode for practising paediatric endocrinologists, as well as the patients they were treating with HGH and their families, started when our LWPES colleagues observed 3 cases of fatal Creutzfeldt-Jakob disease (CJD) in people below the age of 30, which were reported to the US National Institutes of Health (NIH) in the spring of 1985. They had all received cadaveric pituitary HGH, which had been extracted at the National Pituitary Agency (NPA) of the NIH, for treating their severe GH deficiency during the years 1963–1976, two of them with the same batch of HGH. In April 1985 the NPA stopped distributing extractive HGH and this news immediately reached ESPE members.

We wrote carefully worded letters to the parents of our HGH patients, asking them to stop injections for all except the few children who were at severe risk of hypoglycaemia. At that time, late April 1985, biosynthetic HGH had not yet been approved, and was available for children only in a few clinical trials.

---

81 Minutes of Annual Business Meeting, 1986.
82 Minutes of Council Meeting, 14th January 1987, Paris.

The Joint LWPES/ESPE Organising Committee reacted swiftly, adding two 'emergency' sessions on Pituitary GH to the 2nd Joint Meeting in Baltimore on June 23rd and 24th to discuss how to deal with this new, highly worrying situation. In the meantime, Michael Preece in London had reported the first CJD case after extractive HGH produced by the National Hormone and Pituitary Programme (part of the NHS) in the UK. Invited speakers were Dr. C. Gajdusek from the NIH, who received the Nobel prize in 1976 for detecting Kuru disease transmission and who had confirmed CJD by neuropathology in the US patients, and Dr. G. Faich, an epidemiologist at the FDA. The nightmare of an epidemiological catastrophe in possibly thousands of former HGH recipients loomed, and became a real threat when, in the following years, many more CJD cases, some with unusually short incubation periods, were observed in France following treatment with HGH extracted at the Institut Pasteur in Paris. Jean-Claude Job, chairman of ESPE's Working Group on HGH, regularly informed the Council and the membership of the alarming details. At the Annual Meeting in Zaragoza in 1992, a special Round Table on the present situation regarding HGH therapy was held, with updates from the UK (M. Preece) and France (J.C. Job). This resulted in the *Official ESPE Statements on the Safety of HGH*, which was published in 1993.[83] Fortunately, biosynthetic HGH became available for the treatment of GHD children in most European countries after mid-1985.

Fortunately, the worst case scenario did not develop, although up to 2006, 107 cases of CJD after treatment with extractive HGH were counted in France and 51 cases in the UK, with clearly decreasing frequency.[84] It is remarkable that in the other European countries, where the (more expensive) extractive HGH preparations produced by the pharmaceutical industry[85] were used almost exclusively, no CJD cases have been observed to date. One might speculate that the more rigorously controlled purification processes in the industrial setting (e.g. with early use of expensive Sephadex gel chromatography steps) may account for these striking regional differences within Europe.

The CJD/HGH episode taught us (1) to carefully observe and follow our former patients, even as adults (made easier by close long term cooperation with adult endocrinologists) and (2) that carefully controlled, experienced pharmaceutical companies may have a much better quality performance than their public reputation might imply.

In view of this experience, it was clear that the increasing number of children receiving the new recombinant HGH should be subjected to long-term surveillance regarding safety and efficacy, even after the end of treatment. With considerable investment from the HGH-producing companies, many national and international multicentric treatment studies were set up, almost all of them with prominent ESPE members as the main investigators.

---

83 Ritzén EM, et al: Safety of human growth hormone therapy. Horm Res 1993;39:92–93 and following articles, pp 94–110.
84 Brown P, et al: Iatrogenic Creutzfeldt-Jakob disease: the waning of an era. Neurology 2006;67:389–393.
85 Crescormon® by KabiVitrum, Nanormon® by Nordisk, Grorm® by Serono.

The Daily Business of ESPE

In 1983, it was decided to change the membership fee: the annual subscription was increased from SFR 70 to 100, the additional SFR 30 were put into a Joint Meeting account to cover the costs of the Joint Meetings with the LWPES.[86] It was also decided that retired members would no longer have to pay an annual fee – in 1981 a proposal to this effect had been rejected. Since 1990 retired members may make a voluntary contribution of SFR 50 to cover the costs of postage, etc. Since some members from eastern European countries had difficulties paying the annual subscription in 'hard' Western currencies, the Council decided in 1984 to decide on a case by case basis and not to force anybody to pay. In 1987, for the first time, the President-Elect of the forthcoming Annual Meeting attended the Council Meetings as a non-voting Council Member.

In 1987, Karger Publishers offered to make *Hormone Research* the official ESPE journal. This would incur no costs for the ESPE and the advantages would be a reduced subscription charge, free publication of the meeting abstracts and free publication of ESPE announcements. The participants at the Annual Business Meeting expressed concern that *Hormone Research* was not dedicated solely to paediatric endocrinology and was not the best international journal as it had only a small circulation and very long publication times. Moreover, questions of coordination should be clarified in detail in advance, as well as the relationship with *Pediatric Research* regarding the publication of abstracts.

The Council saw a benefit for the Society in this connection if the quality of the journal were improved under a new editorial board involving the ESPE. The majority of the members present were also in favour, and in 1988 the Council elected Milo Zachmann as future associate editor-in-chief. In 1990, the abstracts of the Joint Meeting in Jerusalem in 1989 were published in *Hormone Research*.

In 1989, the International Coordination Office of Pediatric Endocrine Societies (COPES) was founded to coordinate the exchange of information about meetings, courses, fellowships, etc. between the ESPE, the Lawson Wilkins Pediatric Endocrine Society, the Latin American Pediatric Endocrine Society and the Japanese Pediatric Endocrine Society. In 1993, it was re-named as the International Communication Office of Pediatric Endocrine Societies.

---

86 Minutes of Annual Business Meeting, 1983.

The ESPE Tie and Scarf

In 1986, the Secretary Al Aynsley-Green proposed to the Council the introduction of an ESPE tie made by a manufacturer of club ties in England. He planned to buy 100 ties and to recoup the costs when they were sold at the Annual Meeting. The male Council members were in favour and there was opposition only from one female member 'who felt that this initiative reflected an underlying sexist attitude to the female members of the Society.' The Secretary stressed that this had not been behind his suggestion and that he would be happy to investigate the possibility of having a scarf with the ESPE logo made if the female ESPE members wanted this. The scarves were sold out on the first day of the meeting in Zurich and ESPE made an unplanned profit of SFR 400.

In 1995, when Al Aynsley-Green was President of the Edinburgh Annual Meeting, a new ESPE tie was designed and successfully sold there and at subsequent ESPE meetings.

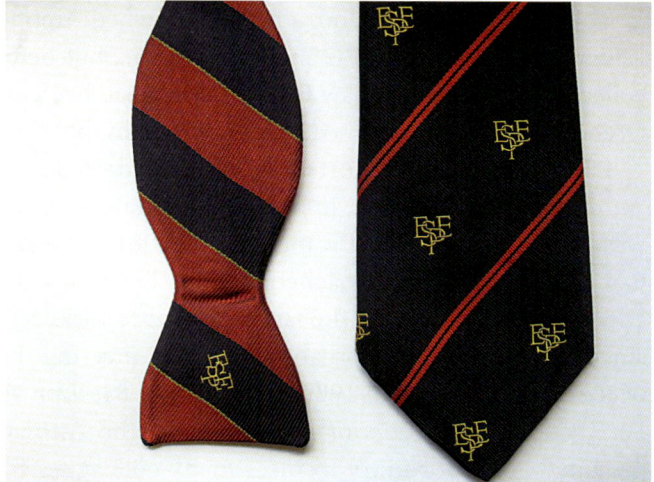

The ESPE ties: left the bow tie from 1995, right the tie from 1986.

Going East – New Members in Central, Eastern and Southern Europe (1990s)

East-West Relationships before 1989

In the summer and winter of 1989 the peaceful revolutions in central and eastern Europe put an end to the division of the European continent which had persisted for four decades. For ESPE, too, a new era dawned. Cooperation between east and west was nothing new for ESPE and its members, but before 1989 only a few privileged colleagues from the Warsaw Pact countries had been allowed to attend scientific conferences such as the ESPE Annual Meetings in the west.

Long before 1989 efforts had been made to organise ESPE Annual Meetings 'behind the Iron Curtain', in order to facilitate scientific exchange between east and west. At the Geneva ESPE meeting in 1981, Al Aynsley-Green and several other Council members approached Ferenc Péter, the leading Hungarian paediatric endocrinologist, head of the largest Budapest children's hospital and ESPE member since 1979, in order to organise an ESPE meeting in Budapest 'to allow inclusion of the Eastern European countries'.[87] In 1983, with the help of the ESPE Council, Feri Péter and his co-workers organised the Annual Meeting in Budapest. This provided an opportunity to meet many colleagues from behind the Iron Curtain. Arrangements were also made to supply eastern European colleagues with current publications, such as *Hormone Research*.[88] The 1991 Annual Meeting with Volker Hesse, one of the leading paediatric endocrinologists in the GDR, as President had been awarded to Berlin by ESPE while the Berlin Wall was still standing, and was intended to promote scientific exchange between the two political hemispheres. By the time the meeting took place the city was re-united, and the Berlin Annual Meeting was organised with the help of the West Berlin colleagues, Bruno Weber and Hans Helge.[89]

---

87 Péter F: Progress in Paediatrica Endocrinology. Budapest Science Press, 2008.
88 Eye witness report W. Sippell; Programme Annual ESPE Meeting, Budapest 1983.
89 Eye witness report W. Sippell.

ESPE Clinical Fellowship, ESPE Winter School and Other Support Programmes

In the 1990s, specific efforts were made to support candidates from the former Warsaw Pact countries. This opening up of ESPE fell during the tenures in office as Secretary of Ieuan Hughes (1987–1992) and Wolfgang Sippell (1992–1997). In 1993, 61 young scientists received travel grants to attend the Joint Meeting in San Francisco, nine of them from Russia, Bulgaria, Poland and the Ukraine.[90] In 1995/1996, the Council agreed 'that for the eastern European applicants the relatively strict criteria for membership cannot be applied as stringently as for other applicants'.[91]

In 1992, at a meeting of the Executive Committee of the European Federation of Endocrine Societies (EFES, now known as the European Society of Endocrinology, ESE), it was agreed to form a Coordination Committee dedicated to the training of young endocrinologists in eastern Europe.[92] However, ESPE was much faster out of the starting block compared with the European adult endocrinologists at EFES, and also more successful; great effort was put into establishing new training programmes to further young colleagues from the eastern European countries and to bring their qualifications up to western European standards. With the Clinical Training Fellowship and the Winter School (postgraduate course), ESPE created two programmes which would help compensate existing deficits.

In 1991, Ares-Serono SA agreed to finance a Clinical Training Fellowship for young eastern European scientists.[93] The requirements for a full-term Clinical Fellowship, lasting from 1 to 2 years, or for a short-term Clinical Fellowship, were the support of the home institute and knowledge in general paediatrics. The host centre receiving the scientist should have an excellent reputation.[94] The Selection Committee comprised three ESPE members, a member of ESPE Council and a representative of the sponsor, Ares-Serono. In 1997, new guidelines were established for the ESPE Clinical Fellowship: from then on there would be a 1-year Clinical Fellowship and a short-term Clinical Fellowship running from 3 to 6 months.[95]

The Winter School was intended to complement the Summer School and was organised in a similar fashion. However, it is not held at the same time as the Annual Meeting, but rather in the winter or spring, in a different central or eastern European country every year. It also has a fundamentally different focus. The Winter School was set up with the aim of imparting basic knowledge of paediatric endocrinology. A Steering Committee was established which could concentrate on the particular problems of the young Eastern European scientists. The prevailing opinion at the first

---

90 Minutes of Annual Business Meeting, 1993.
91 Minutes of Council Meeting, 26th–27th April, 1996, Montpellier; cf. Minutes of Council Meeting, 14th November, 1995, Montpellier.
92 Minutes of Annual Business Meeting, 1992.
93 ESPE archives, letter from J.-P. Bourguignon, 12th July 1991; 'ESPE Clinical Fellowship sponsored by Serono'.
94 Minutes of Annual Business Meeting, 1991.
95 Minutes of Annual Business Meeting, 1997.

Winter School Teachers' Meeting was 'that the basic medical school background was not as elaborate as in western Europe'.[96]

The first Winter School (postgraduate course) was held December 8th–12th 1995 in Seregélyes near Lake Balaton in Hungary, with Ze'ev Hochberg acting as coordinator. The participants came from Hungary, Slovenia, Croatia, the Czech Republic and Slovakia (see figure on p. 92). In fact, the candidates turned out to be much better qualified than expected. The Steering Committee stated: 'All participants agreed that the level of the students was higher than anticipated with very good case presentations'.[97] The Ferring company, which had already been supporting the Summer School financially for many years, agreed to sponsor the Winter School to the annual sum of USD 25,000.[98] From 1996 on, the supervisors from the students' home institutions were also invited to attend as 'senior mentors'. The idea behind this was to improve acceptance of the ESPE Winter School among the Winter School students' superiors, while at the same time breaking down barriers.[99]

One topic which greatly preoccupied the ESPE as well as the Winter School participants during these years was age- and child-friendly methods of examination.[100] Ethical standards in paediatric endocrinological research were also discussed. As already mentioned, these subjects had been under discussion in the Society in the 1980s, but now it became particularly evident that the ideas on ethics in the different European countries diverged widely. Many of the abstracts submitted to the 1992 Annual Meeting in Zaragoza did not meet ESPE requirements but 'were raising ethical problems for all participants'.[101]

Both programmes, the Clinical Fellowship and the Winter School, were extremely successful. A Council Meeting in 1996 came to the conclusion that the first Winter School 'had been a very valuable experience for all concerned'.[102]

The ESPE Visiting Scholarship, financed by Kabi Pharmacia, was another ESPE project which supported young eastern European academics from 1993 on. With an easy, one page application form, it enabled ESPE members' young co-workers who were involved in an ongoing research project, to make a short visit to a laboratory, generally in Western Europe, to learn or improve methods needed for the project.

---

96 Various problems were discussed: diagnostic shortcomings, poor English, lack of modern lab equipment, uncritical use of untested drugs – the faculty wanted to emphasize the importance of accurate dosage and pass on standardised monitoring methods. Cf. W. Sippell, Z. Hochberg: Postgraduate Course (Winter School) Minutes of Teachers' Meeting for course to be held in Hungary from 8th–12th December, 1995.

97 Cf. W. Sippell, Z. Hochberg: Postgraduate Course (Winter School) Minutes of Teachers' Meeting for course to be held in Hungary from 8th–12th December, 1995.

98 ESPE archives, letter from C. Thomas (Managing Director, Ferring Arzneimittel GmbH) to W. Sippell, 23th January, 1995.

99 Cf. ESPE archives. Letter from Z. Hochberg to Steering Committee: Progress Report, 17th April, 1996; eye witness report W. Sippell.

100 Minutes of Winter School Steering Committee Meeting, 12th December, 1995, Seregélyes (Hungary).

101 Minutes of Council Meeting, 12th May, 1992, Rotterdam; Eye witness report W. Sippell.

102 Minutes of Council Meeting, 15th September, 1996, Montpellier.

The knowledge thus acquired should result in improved research at the fellow's home laboratory.[103]

In 1999, the ESPE Annual Meeting was held in Warsaw with Tomasz Romer from the Children's Memorial Health Institute in Warsaw as President. The Secretary reported: 'This meeting [. . .] was an outstanding success. There were over 1,300 delegates and the Opera House was brilliantly converted to a highly attractive and functional venue.'[104] At this meeting participants found it difficult to believe that Europe had been divided for so many years, and this was even less evident at the more recent ESPE meetings in Ljubljana 2003 and in Prague in 2010.

New Members

The fall of the Iron Curtain and the opening of ESPE to the east resulted in a significant increase in membership numbers. In the 1980s there had been, on average, 13–14 new members a year, and from the mid-1990s this increased to 20–30, and in 1996 44 new members were admitted. A quarter of these were from the former Eastern Bloc countries.[105] Prior to this the greatest increase had been in 1989 when 52 new members had been accepted; however, 'the large number of applications in 1989 was due to the dropping of the former long-standing rule that applications should lie on the table for one year'.[106] The ESPE membership more than doubled between 1988 (254 members) and 1999 (520 members).

In 1993, the annual membership fee, which was now being collected in Dutch guilders (Sten Drop, Rotterdam had been elected as new Treasurer), was increased for the first time in 10 years by about 15% to 150 guilders.[107] Since the costs of the now much more diverse Society had increased and the balance only remained positive thanks to profits made at previous Annual Meetings, the membership fee was increased again in 1994 by NLG 50. The eastern European members did not have to pay this fee in full, or at all, if they could not afford it.[108]

Scientific Standards and Greater Differentiation

The assurance and improvement of scientific standards also played a central role in ESPE in the 1990s. By this time the abstracts submitted for the Annual Meeting were

---

103 Minutes of Annual Business Meeting, 1993.
104 Secretary's Annual Report, 2000.
105 Minutes of Annual Business Meeting, 1996.
106 Minutes of Council Meeting, 26th–27th April 1996, Montpellier.
107 Minutes of Council Meeting, 26th–27th April 1996, Montpellier.
108 Minutes of Annual Business Meeting, 1994.

being systematically evaluated 'in blind fashion', based on a clear scoring system[109] and divided into topics.[110] A questionnaire was also distributed to the members in an effort to ensure that the contents of the Annual Meetings were better adapted to the members' needs.[111]

An important step was taken in 1992, at the suggestion of Al Aynsley-Green and Ralph Rappaport, with the setting up of a Programme Organising Committee (POC). This had been proposed several times since the mid-1980s,[112] to ensure that every relevant topic was covered in depth in the long term. This had not always been the case. In 1988, two senior members wrote to Council: 'We are writing you on a rather serious matter which concerns the quality of a number of papers presented at the meeting of ESPE. We are very worried by the at best very mediocre quality of some papers presented in the sections on growth and allied subjects. [...] To explain the disappointing quality we would hate to think that this represents the standard of performance of the present members and guests of the ESPE; we prefer to assume that the referee system followed by the ESPE is not sufficiently rigid. [...] Moreover, the increasing diversity and intricacy of the subjects covered at recent meetings renders selection of papers more difficult than it was in the earlier days of the ESPE'.[113]

Following these comments, demands were made for a Planning Committee to be set up, and for its existence to be anchored in the constitution.[114] Following extensive discussions this was acted on in 1992.

The main task of the Advisory POC, which comprised 12 people chosen from among the Council and the Summer School Steering Committee members, was the long-term planning of subjects to be covered at the Annual Scientific Meetings. It also played a liaison role between the different annual Presidents. The Executive POC, comprising the President, the Secretary and two or three other members, was responsible for the more detailed planning. Ralph Rappaport was elected as first chairman of the Advisory POC.[115]

Different working groups had come into being since the early 1980s. The Working Party on Congenital hypothyroidism was set up in 1979/80[116] and the Working Party

109 Minutes of Council Meeting, 6th–7th June, 1990, Vienna.
110 Cf. Minutes of Council Meeting, 3rd May, 1989, Paris; Minutes of Council Meeting, 2nd February 1990, Amsterdam.
111 Minutes of Council Meeting 2nd–3rd May, 1991, Berlin.
112 Minutes of Council Meeting 2nd September 1984, Heidelberg. A 'Charter for the President' was also proposed. Cf. Minutes of Council Meeting, June 1985, Baltimore.
113 ESPE archives, letter from M. Preece/R. Steendijk to ESPE Council, 2nd November, 1987.
114 ESPE archives, letter from M. Preece/R. Steendijk to ESPE Council, 2nd November, 1987.
115 Cf. Comments on proposal from Aynsley-Green, Minutes of Council Meeting, 6th–7th June, 1990, Vienna; Minutes of Council Meeting, 2nd September 1990, Vienna; ESPE archives, letter from W. Sippell to A. Aynsley-Green, 9th October 1992; Minutes of Annual Business Meeting, 1992.
116 ESPE Working Group on Congenital Hypothyroidism: Guidelines for Neonatal Screening Programs for Congenital Hypothyroidism. Grüters A, Delange F, Giovanelli G, Klett M, Rochiccioli P, Torresani T, Grant D, Hnikova O, Mäenpää J, Rondanini GF, Toublanc JE: Horm Res 1994;41:1–2.

on the Use of Human Growth Hormone was established in 1984 to address the safety problems of HGH therapy.[117] The latter prepared official ESPE statements for publication in 1993[118] and acted as an advisory committee to Council. In the following year it was decided that the Working Group should be reorganised as the Drugs and Therapeutics Committee (DTC).[119] The committee should meet twice a year and liaise with the LWPES Drugs and Therapeutics Committee.[120] Other working groups were involved with the pan-European Diagnostic Classification Project (from 1993) and Neonatal Screening (from 1995).[121]

From 1997 ESPE formed a subsection of the Confederation of European Societies in Paediatrics (CESP) and thus became a member of the European Board of Paediatrics (EBP), which works to establish standards of training in paediatrics. The EBP asked the ESPE to take responsibility for paediatric endocrinology in Europe and to set up an Education and Training Subcommittee.[122]

Facilitating Research

A number of research programmes were established or developed further in the 1990s in addition to the programmes aimed specifically at improving paediatric endocrinology in eastern and central Europe.

ESPE Sabbatical Leave Programme

The Sabbatical Leave Programme was introduced in 1993. It enables senior ESPE members to leave their home institute to carry out research in another institute for a year. The programme offers the recipient a unique opportunity for scientific renewal, new research development and the establishment of collaborative links. Eli Lilly agreed to finance this programme.[123]

---

117 Minutes of Annual Business Meeting, 1980, 1984.
118 Ritzén EM, et al: Safety of human growth hormone therapy. Horm Res 1993;39:92–93 and following articles, pp 94–110.
119 Minutes of Annual Business Meeting, 1991.
120 From 1993, the DTC focussed on following topics: growth hormone related issues, notably CJD and leukaemia, drugs in sport, hormone-containing local applications, topical corticosteroids, hormone preparation in limited supply in certain countries, insulin and pumps and the role of cyclosporin in diabetes. Cf. Minutes of Annual Business Meeting, 1992.
121 Minutes of Council Meeting, 1993; Minutes of Council Meeting, 1995.
122 Minutes of Annual Business Meeting, 1997.
123 Minutes of Annual Business Meeting, 1993.

ESPE Young Investigator Award

The Young Investigator Award, a prize for young European paediatric endocrinologists below the age of 40, was instigated in 1993 with the support of the Swedish-based company Pharmacia. This prize, worth SEK 25,000, has since been awarded almost every year for excellent, peer-reviewed scientific publications.[124]

ESPE Research Award

In 1995 a new Senior Investigator Award, the ESPE Research Award, which is also financed by Pharmacia, Stockholm, was set up. It is intended to close the gap between the Young Investigator Award for young scientists under 40 and the Andrea Prader Prize for senior members. The award, which is worth SEK 40,000, is given to ESPE members in recognition of scientific work which has made an important contribution to paediatric endocrinology.[125] The recipients of the Young Investigator and Research Awards are selected by the Andrea Prader Prize Committee.

Outstanding Clinician Award

The Outstanding Clinician Award was established in 2001, again with the support of Pharmacia, Stockholm, and is awarded annually to an ESPE member in recognition of outstanding contributions to the practice of clinical paediatric endocrinology. The recipient receives 20.000 SEK and a certificate. Candidates should be proposed by two ESPE members, the Andrea Prader Prize Committee selects the winner.[126]

The Young Investigator Award, the Research Award, the Outstanding Clinician Award and the Andrea Prader Prize are now financed by the US pharma group Pfizer, which bought up Pharmacia in 2002.

---

124 Minutes of Annual Business Meeting, 1993.
125 Minutes of Annual Business Meeting, 1995.
126 Minutes of Annual Business Meeting, 2000.

ESPE Evolves

Annual Meetings: Challenges and Changes

As a result of the work of the new Programme Organising Committee (POC), the format of the Annual Meetings was further modified in the 1990s. In 1993, Ralph Rappaport, the Chairman of the POC, developed guidelines for the organisation of the Annual Meetings which should apply for all POC members and future Presidents. Here the purpose of the Annual Meetings was clearly defined: 'to provide state of the art communication on controversial, complex and rapidly advancing issues. In view of the large and quite varied experience of the many members of ESPE, it is also important to offer the best opportunities for presenting members' own research data in all areas. In addition, ESPE members should be exposed to current medical and scientific knowledge in all areas which may be relevant to developmental, biological and medical progress'.[127]

Rappaport pointed out that 'apart from the symposia and plenary lectures, poster and oral presentations are the active core of any meeting'.[128] The coexistence of these different types of events should enable young scientists to become more involved in the discussion process, 'thus fostering European exchange and collaboration'.[129] At the same time, particular attention should be paid to ensuring that the scientific standard of the meetings was in accordance with clearly defined criteria. The guidelines stated: 'An important issue is the choice of the main speakers. [. . .] Owing to the high standard of our Society, we have been able to attract top scientists and clinicians from all over the world, and there should, therefore, be no difficulty in being appropriately selective in the future.'[130]

---

127 R. Rappaport: The ESPE Programme Organising Committee (POC), attached to letter from W. Sippell to members of the Programme Organising Committee, 27th April 1993.
128 R. Rappaport: The ESPE Programme Organising Committee (POC), attached to letter from W. Sippell to members of the Programme Organising Committee, 27th April 1993.
129 R. Rappaport: The ESPE Programme Organising Committee (POC), attached to letter from W. Sippell to members of the Programme Organising Committee, 27th April 1993.
130 R. Rappaport: The ESPE Programme Organising Committee (POC), attached to letter from W. Sippell to members of the Programme Organising Committee, 27th April 1993.

With the wide variety of scientific contributions, many members felt there was a need for more expert moderation with regard to content. Steven Shalet revived the idea of guided poster tours in 1995, when he drafted special guidelines for tour leaders.[131] At the 36th Annual Meeting in Stockholm in 1997, mini-poster sessions on selected topics were held for the first time in addition to the guided tours. Medical controversy workshops provided a new framework for discussing specific disputed diagnostic and therapeutic problems. Sessions on clinical research methods were also introduced.

In 1999, clinical practice sessions were established and held as parallel sessions. They preceded the later 'Meet the Expert' sessions. A sense of competition between basic science on the one hand and clinical practice on the other again became apparent in the Annual Meeting programmes; the ESPE POC was eager to achieve a balance between these two poles.

Further specialisation within the field of paediatric endocrinology resulted in more changes to the overall structure of the Annual Meetings: Since 2003, new ESPE speciality clubs and study groups, such as the 'Bone Club', the 'Obesity Club' and the Working Groups on Turner syndrome, growth plate, disorders of sex development (DSD) and paediatric and adolescent gynaecology (PAG) meet before the official opening of the Meeting.

Other changes were also made. In 1997, the last full-day excursion was arranged as an official part of the social programme and included in the registration fee: an unforgettable boat cruise through the Stockholm archipelago with beautiful midsummer weather. This 35-year-old ESPE tradition had to be sacrificed to the ever-increasing number of participants and to the need not to extend the overall duration of the annual meeting to more than 4 days.

A More Professional Approach

In view of the growing numbers of participants at the Annual Meetings – there were, for the first time, more than one thousand registrations for the 35th Annual Meeting in Montpellier in 1996[132] – and the insecurity with regard to regular funding[133], from the mid-1990s a fundamental debate developed on the organisation

---

131 ESPE archives, letter from S.M. Shalet to W. Sippell: Guided poster tours, cf. ESPE archives, answering letter from W. Sippell to S.M. Shalet, 21st December, 1995.

132 ESPE archives, letter from S.M. Shalet to W. Sippell: Guided poster tours, cf. ESPE archives, answering letter from W. Sippell to S.M. Shalet, 21st December, 1995.

133 'Financial liability for ESPE Annual Meetings'. As already discussed under item 3b, the ESPE cannot yet take on financial liability for the Annual Meetings. Therefore, for the time being, each President will have to tackle the problem on a national basis'. Minutes of Council Meeting, 27th–28th October 1994, London; cf. ESPE archives, letter from A. Aynsley-Green to W. Sippell, S. Drop, 9th April, 1996.

of meetings and the 'future structure of ESPE'.[134] The focus was on finding ways to increase revenue to a level comparable with other major scientific organisations. A further increase in the membership fees was debated, the idea of obtaining money from the pharmaceutical industry for financing the Annual Meetings or of employing a professional organising consultant were considered, as was the idea of setting up a permanent ESPE Secretariat. Notwithstanding the controversial discussions, there was agreement on the common 'goal of organising the Society and the Annual Meetings more professionally in future'.[135]

With the Secretary overseeing the project, work had been started on compiling a President's Handbook in 1996/1997,[136] and the suggestions drawn up by Leo Van den Brande were particularly helpful in this respect.[137] In 2000, the Programme Organising Committee decided to continue with this project 'as it was felt important that the details which are currently being learnt about the organisation of the Annual ESPE Meeting should be written down and used for future Presidents'.[138]

In this way ESPE was endeavouring to bridge the gap between the small, family-like scientific organisation which the long-standing members had known and the greatly expanded, differentiated international society it has become. In the Annual Report in 1997, the Secretary drew the following résumé:

'In its 36th year, in terms of membership numbers, ESPE is still one of the smaller paediatric subspecialty societies in Europe, but in terms of scientific achievements and training activities it is certainly one of the most active. Although, as my predecessor Ieuan Hughes pointed out, ESPE is no longer the small family-like club of European paediatric endocrinologists of its early days, it is still small enough to enable international scientific cooperation on a personal level'.[139]

Congrex

A major step towards putting the Annual Meetings on a more professional and safe footing was taken when ESPE hired, for the first time in 1996/1997, the services of the Swedish conference organiser, Congrex Stockholm. This was even more important in view of the painful experience with the previous congress organising company 'Chairman' in Montpellier who, after the meeting, 'disappeared with all

---

134 Minutes of Council Meeting, 14th November, 1995, Montpellier; cf. answering letter, M.O. Savage to P. Chatelain, 5th June 1995; '15. Discussion with past Presidents, Dr. Aynsley-Green and Dr. Van den Brande', in: Confidential appendix to Minutes of Council Meeting, 15th September 1996, Montpellier.
135 Minutes of Council Meeting, 14th November 1995, Montpellier.
136 ESPE archives, letter from W. Sippell to L. Van den Brande, 3rd July 1996; ESPE archives, letter from W. Sippell to C. Sultan, ESPE President's Handbook, 22nd January, 1997.
137 ESPE archives, letter L. Van den Brande to W. Sippell: Organising the ESPE meetings – suggestions for future Presidents. 7 pages including time table, 29th January, 1997.
138 Minutes of Programme Organising Committee Meeting, 2000.
139 Secretary's Annual Report, 1997.

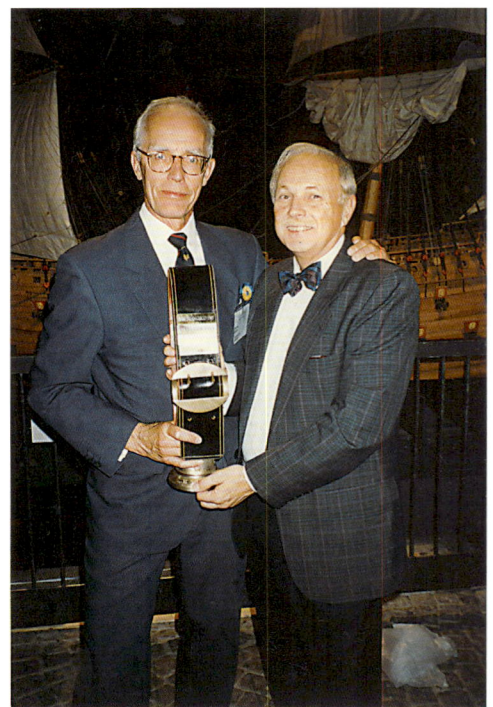

Pierre Sizonenko (right) presents the Swiss Joint Meeting Bell to Martin Ritzén (left) at the opening of the 5th Joint Meeting in Stockholm, 1997.

the charts and 1 Million French francs (EUR 150,000)'.[140] Congrex, in contrast, had successfully organised conferences for various international scientific organisations and was able to provide services which covered project management, finances, registration of participants and hotel bookings, as well as helping to organise the social events. A particular advantage was Congrex's expertise in processing the abstracts electronically.[141] In 1998, a 2-year contract was agreed with Congrex to organise the meetings in 1999 in Warsaw and in 2000 in Brussels.[142] During this time the system of abstract rating and the design of the abstract forms were further improved and, thanks to the technical back-up from Congrex, the work of the POC became more efficient.[143] Council was extremely pleased with the organisation of the mini-poster

---

140 E-mail from C. Sultan to W. Sippell, 1st June, 2011.
141 Cf. Congrex: Proposal for the annual congress of the European Society for Paediatric Endocrinology, Stockholm, 9th May, 1997.
142 Minutes of Council Meeting, 24th September, 1998, Florence.
143 'Dr. Ritzen commented favourably on the workings of the Mini POC. This worked extremely efficiently when the meeting was held in the Congrex Offices as computer backup was present, which facilitated the arrangements.' Minutes of Council Meeting, 7th–8th May, 1999, London.

symposia in Warsaw: 'the quality of these sessions looked excellent'.[144] Following the successful organisation of the meetings in Warsaw and Brussels, the Council signed a 4-year contract with Congrex.[145] As a result of the good cooperation this contract was further extended,[146] so that Congrex is still the professional organiser for the ESPE Annual Meetings.

Agreements with the Pharmaceutical Industry

Cooperation with the sponsors from the pharmaceutical industry, which was becoming ever more regulated, was also important for ensuring a professional approach to the Annual Meetings in the coming years. Agreements were reached on opportunities for pharmaceutical companies to present themselves during the meetings and on financial support.

In 1995, the Council agreed to more extensive acknowledgement of the sponsors in the Annual Meeting programme and 'that sponsorship of ESPE Awards, Fellowships and Educational programmes by pharmaceutical companies should be acknowledged on one or two extra pages in the final programme of the Annual Meeting, and that sponsoring companies should be mentioned within the programme – as was done in Edinburgh 1995 – without asking for Council's or POC agreement'.[147] In the following year, however, in line with the already prevailing attitude in ESPE, the Council members decided that pharmaceutical companies should not sponsor individual sessions or symposia.[148] In 1998, the Secretary entered into negotiations with various pharmaceutical companies 'concerning a new longer term financial arrangement for supporting the Annual Meeting'.[149] Agreement on this was reached in 1999: The five major sponsors at the time, Eli Lilly, Ferring, Novo Nordisk, Pharmacia and Serono, guaranteed fixed sums for supporting the Annual Meeting. A meeting was arranged with representatives of these companies during the Annual Meeting.[150] In the following years, new agreements were made with additional sponsors.[151]

In 2003, following controversial discussions in Council, a limited number of industry-sponsored Satellite symposia were permitted during the Annual Meetings.[152] The new task of evaluating the content and selecting the Satellite meetings was trans-

144   Dr. Ritzen commented favourably on the workings of the Mini POC. This worked extremely efficiently when the meeting was held in the Congrex Offices as computer backup was present, which facilitated the arrangements.' Minutes of Council Meeting, 7th–8th May, 1999, London.
145   Secretary's Annual Report, 2001.
146   Minutes of Council Meeting, 10th September 2004, Basel.
147   Minutes of Council Meeting, 14th November, 1995, Montpellier.
148   Minutes of Council Meeting, 15th September, 1996, Montpellier.
149   Minutes of Council Meeting, 24th September, 1998, Florence.
150   Minutes of Council Meeting, 7th–8th May, 1999, London; Secretary's Annual Report, 2000.
151   Cf. e.g. Minutes of Council Meeting, 16th September, 2000, Brussels.
152   Minutes of Council Meeting, 17th September, 2003, Ljubljana.

ferred to the POC in 2005. The Minutes of the Council Meeting recorded that: 'the satellites were a success, but programmes should be submitted to the POC for approval eight months before the meeting in future'.[153]

In the same year the Corporate Liaison Board (CLB), with the ESPE Secretary Martin Savage as Chairperson, was set up 'to serve as a forum for regular and direct two-way communication between ESPE and Paediatric Endocrinology in industry'.[154] The CLB also works to increase the number of sponsors. Three levels of sponsors for the Annual Meetings were introduced (platinum, gold, silver) in order to attract more companies. The CLB is made up of ESPE members, representatives of the platinum sponsors, Congrex and Bioscientifica (the ESPE secretariat in Bristol).[155]

New Priorities, New Structures

Over the last two decades ESPE has grown into an organisation which covers very diverse activities. New responsibilities and important services have been taken on and new committees established in which forward-looking decisions have been taken on behalf of paediatric endocrinology, since the end of the 1990s in the fields of training/education and clinical practice in particular. Against this backdrop, in 2003 the Society again underwent internal restructuring, in order to reflect the priorities and the current state of ESPE activities.

Strategic Planning and New Management

There were radical innovations with regard to organisation and management. During the Annual Business Meeting in 2001, it was decided to set up a Strategic Planning Committee (SPC) 'which would consider a number of key areas related to the organisation within ESPE'.[156] The first Chairperson of this committee was Stephen Shalet and its main task was to 'review organisational procedures within ESPE'.[157] These included the organisation of the Secretariat and monitoring the workload, efficiency and finances. The new committee 'would seek the opinion of the membership on key areas such as identification of major future challenges for ESPE'[158] and should report to Council. It was also responsible for maintaining the ESPE website.

Soon after its founding, the SPC started work on developing an appropriate concept for internal change. The ESPE Secretariat was restructured in 2003. Up till then

---

153 Minutes of Council Meeting, 7th–8th January, 2005, Brussels.
154 Minutes of Annual Business Meeting, 2005.
155 Minutes of Annual Business Meeting, 2005.
156 Minutes of Annual Business Meeting, 2001.
157 Minutes of Annual Business Meeting, 2001.
158 Minutes of Annual Business Meeting, 2001.

the Secretaries had dealt with ESPE administration within their University departments. ESPE supported them in this by financing a part time secretarial assistant and reimbursing major office expenses.

However, with the growth of ESPE and the increasing number of tasks involved, a new form of management became necessary. The organization of the ESPE office was transferred to BioScientifica in Bristol. BioScientifica is a commercial subsidiary of the (British) Society for Endocrinology, and has taken over the administration of several other scientific organisations which focus on endocrinology.[159]

Key Committees and Changes in Council

Following the SPC proposals several so-called Key Committees were established – in addition to the POC these were a Finance Committee (FC), an Education and Training Committee (ETC) and a Clinical Practice Committee (CPC).[160]

The Chairpersons of the different Key Committees should have a seat in Council and stand for election at the Business Meeting. Council should also include two members with no responsibility in a Key Committee. This draft proposal and the amendments were put before the Business Meeting in Madrid in 2002, and 'strongly approved by the Membership'.[161]

This new structure was an important step towards making ESPE 'more compatible with the modern academic requirements of teaching, research and patient care'.[162] The personal link between the key Committees and Council resulted in a more effective division of labour. The Secretary was relieved of some of his workload, and a greater degree of internal democracy and participation of ESPE members in the key areas of the organisation was achieved. In his Annual Report in 2003, Secretary Francesco Chiarelli wrote: 'Following the positive vote to change the constitution to allow wider representation in Council and the development of Key Committees, and also to lighten the load of the General Secretary, the Chairs of the POC, Training Committee and Clinical Practice Committee will be democratically voted at the Business Meeting in Basel. According to the constitution, the new Chairs will be members of Council.'[163]

---

159 Secretary's Annual Report, 2004; Minutes of Annual Business Meeting, 2004.
160 Minutes of Council Meeting, 12th December, 2002, Ljubljana.
161 Secretary's Annual Report, 2003. The amendment read: 'The Society should be governed by a Council consisting of 7 ordinary members. The General Secretary and Chairs of the Finance Committee, Training Committee, Programme Organising Committee and Clinical Practice Committee will hold these positions for 3 years with the possibility of re-election for one further term of 3 years.' See Minutes of Council Meeting, 12th December, 2002, Ljubljana.
162 Secretary's Annual Report, 2003.
163 Secretary's Annual Report, 2004.

Publications and Information

At the same time a more professional approach was also taken to information and communication in ESPE. The ESPE homepage went online in 1998,[164] and was further upgraded in 2005.[165] In 2004, the Newsletter Editorial Board designed a new ESPE Newsletter to provide space for addressing specific issues in detail. ESPE's aim with this newsletter is 'to build up a sense of community among European paediatric endocrinologists, with a view of strengthening the discipline and increasing ESPE membership'.[166] It is mailed electronically, is generally 4–8 pages long and is sent to all members as well as to all important contacts. Ipsen Biopharmaceuticals agreed to finance the newsletter.[167] *Hormone Research* has been the official ESPE Journal since 1989.[168] Experienced ESPE members have served as Editors-in-Chief: Jürg Girard (Basel) 1976–1995, Michael Ranke (Tübingen) 1996–2003[169], and since 2004 Paul Czernichow (Paris).[170] In 2005 *Hormone Research* introduced some new features (mini-reviews, novel insights from clinical experience) and the contract with the publisher S. Karger, Basel, Switzerland, was extended. In January 2010, the Journal was renamed *Hormone Research in Paediatrics* and is now also the official Journal of ESPE's Latin American sister society, SLEP.

As the body of knowledge in paediatric endocrinology – as in most medical specialties – is expanding very quickly, it has become almost impossible to follow all relevant advances in detail. Therefore, since 2004, the most significant peer-reviewed publications are presented by experts on the topic in question at the Annual Meeting during the so-called 'Yearbook of Paediatric Endocrinology' sessions which are usually extremely well attended. They also appear in book form as commented abstracts: The *Yearbook of Paediatric Endocrinology*, which is endorsed by ESPE, is published by Karger annually. The Yearbook keeps paediatric endocrinologists, paediatricians and endocrinologists informed about new research developments in their field.

Education and Training Committee

The purpose of the Education and Training Committee (ETC), which was established in 2003, is 'to consolidate and promote education and training, for paediatricians in training as well as for continuous medical education (CME) in Paediatric Endocrinology'.[171] Since ESPE activities are increasingly focusing on education and

---

164 Minutes of Council Meeting, 24th September, 1998, Florence.
165 Secretary's Annual Report, 2005.
166 Secretary's Annual Report, 2005.
167 Secretary's Annual Report, 2005.
168 Minutes of Council Meeting, 26th June 1988, Copenhagen and 3rd May, 1989, Paris.
169 Horm Res 1996;46:1.
170 Horm Res 2004;61:2.
171 Secretary's Annual Report, 2010.

training, it was particularly beneficial to combine the various programmes and initiatives under the auspices of one committee. Its key tasks are the organisation and advancement of the Summer and Winter Schools and the establishment of a training centre for paediatric endocrinology in Europe.[172] In 2004, on the initiative of Ze'ev Hochberg and ESPE Council, the programme 'Paediatric Endocrinology in Developing Countries' was launched.[173] Since then, ESPE has been active world-wide in training and education.

Clinical Practice Committee and Consensus Statements

The clinical care of children with endocrine diseases must be ensured and improved, and over the past decade the area of clinical practice has emerged as an important field of activity for ESPE. The committee responsible for overseeing this is the Clinical Practice Committee (CPC), set up in 2003 and chaired by Stefano Cianfarani.[174] The CPC compiles clinical and technical reports and clinical practice guidelines, develops web pages for parents and supports collaborative EU grant applications.[175] The drafting of various Consensus Statements was extremely important for clinical practice and necessitated cooperation with other organisations. The ESPE and the CPC closely cooperate with the LWPES and the GRS (Growth Hormone Research Society).

In 1998, the first GH Research Society/ESPE Consensus Workshop was held on the Diagnosis and Treatment of Adults with GH Deficiency, followed by Consensus Guidelines for the Diagnosis and Treatment of Growth Hormone (GH) Deficiency in Childhood and Adolescence (2000). Since then Consensus Meetings have been held on 'key areas of clinical paediatric endocrinology'.[176] In 2002, the first LWPES/ESPE Consensus Workshop on Congenital Adrenal Hyperplasia was held. To date, Consensus Statements have been adopted on 21-hydroxylase deficiency, diabetic ketoacidosis (DKA), transition care of the GH-treated adolescent, Care of the Intersex Patient, Management of the child born small for gestational age through to adulthood, Use of insulin pump therapy in children, Idiopathic short stature, use of GnRH analogs in children and Insulin resistance in children. For 2011, a Joint Consensus Meeting of representatives of ESPE, LWPES and ISPAD is planned on the subject of 'The Use of Continuous Glucose Sensors (CGS) in the Pediatric Age Group'.[177]

---

172 Secretary's Annual Report, 2005.
173 Secretary's Annual Report, 2005.
174 Secretary's Annual Report, 2010.
175 Secretary's Annual Report, 2005.
176 Secretary's Annual Report, 2004.
177 Secretary's Annual Report, 2010.

Leading World-Wide

Discussions about the Society's Future

At the end of the 1990s, ESPE was flourishing, and enjoyed great international prestige for its scientific achievements. It was on the threshold between being a European society and becoming a scientific organisation with international influence and universal repute. This was also reflected in the international composition of the registrations for the Annual Meetings and in the provenance of the membership applications. Against this background a new debate on the future of ESPE as an organisation was sparked. In which direction should ESPE be heading? What sort of organisation should it become in the new millennium? Questions about further opening up the meetings, and ESPE itself, came to the fore. Should scientists who were not from Europe or the countries bordering on the Mediterranean be allowed to apply for full membership?

One Member – One Guest?

In 1998, the one member-one guest rule for the Annual Meetings gave rise to discussion. Martin Savage, Secretary from 1997 to 2004, concluded in the Council that this rule 'was no longer applicable and discriminatory to basic scientists, scientists outside ESPE countries and other paediatric endocrinologists who would attend the meeting but did not have contact with members'.[178] Savage called for the Annual Meetings to be opened up to participants internationally. He saw the great interest accorded to the Annual Meetings by scientists from all over the world as an indication of ESPE's great success. ESPE's aim should be to become the world leader in the field of paediatric endocrinology. The Minutes of the Council Meeting record: 'The fact that abstracts have been received from Australia, South America and the United States confirmed

---

[178] Minutes of Council Meeting, 24th September, 1998, Florence.

the status of the ESPE meeting as probably the best paediatric endocrine meeting in the world.'[179]

The Secretary suggested that this question should be discussed at the Business Meeting and received Council's approval for this.[180] The discussion at the next Business Meeting showed that the members were fundamentally willing to open up the Annual Meeting more, 'but not yet ready to open the meeting completely without restriction'.[181] In 1999, the amendment to the constitution was voted on, but the proposal to drop the one member-one guest rule did not achieve the necessary two-thirds majority.[182]

The Test Case

In 2000, Dr. Maryam Razzaghy-Azar, a candidate from Iran who had already attended many Annual Meetings, applied for ESPE membership for the first time. Savage spoke on behalf of accepting the Iranian doctor's application. Council finally agreed, but stressed that her election would represent a test case. There were differences of opinion at the Annual Business Meeting; several participants pointed out that it was not possible to accept a candidate from Iran since, according to the constitution, 'Ordinary members shall be appointed from Europe and the Mediterranean'.[183] 84 of the 173 members present agreed that an exception should be made in Dr. Razzaghy-Azar's case, 53 voted against.[184] Following the Annual Business Meeting, however, the topic remained an issue of debate so that Council finally declared the election invalid for formal reasons. Shortly after, following an amendment to the constitution, Dr. Razzaghy-Azar was indeed accepted as the first ESPE member from outside Europe and the Mediterranean countries.[185]

Opening Up of the ESPE

At the Annual Business Meeting in 2001, a paper which Council had received from Leo Van den Brande in May 2000 was discussed. It contained statements from 10 former ESPE Presidents and four former Secretaries with their ideas on the future development of ESPE. The criteria for membership should remain strict 'to keep the scientific exchange between experts in a prominent position in the Annual Meetings'.[186]

179   Minutes of Council Meeting, 24th September, 1998, Florence.
180   Minutes of Council Meeting, 24th September, 1998, Florence.
181   Minutes of Annual Business Meeting, 1998.
182   Minutes of Annual Business Meeting, 1999.
183   Constitution and Regulations [. . .]. Revised [. . .] 28th Annual Meeting, Jerusalem, 1989.
184   Minutes of Annual Business Meeting, 2000.
185   Pers. Recoll., Martin Savage, pp. 111–114 in this book.
186   Minutes of Annual Business Meeting, 2001.

Registration for the Annual Meeting should, however, be opened up. They also warned that the increasing role which was now played by industry in financing the Annual Meetings could lead to a situation of dependency.[187]

In 2001, the Council submitted a proposal to the members to amend the constitution regarding the admission of new members. In future, the relevant section should read as follows: 'Ordinary Members should be appointed from Europe and the Mediterranean. Exceptionally, a candidate from outside this area may be considered for membership on individual merit.' A clear majority was in favour of such a change,[188] so that the statutory basis was now established for accepting candidates from outside Europe. Finally, in 2002, 123 members voted in favour of dropping the one member-one guest rule, so that the appropriate article could be removed from the constitution.[189]

During the Business Meeting in Lyon in 2005 a further change was made to the constitution to facilitate the inclusion of non-European members. Proposals had been made in advance of the meeting by the Council and various senior ESPE members.[190] In his Annual Report the Secretary wrote to the members: 'This year 40 applications have been assessed to be satisfactory by Council. These include further candidates from outside European and Mediterranean countries. With this in mind, a proposal will be discussed at the Business Meeting in Lyon to remove the word "exceptionally" from article 2 of the constitution in regard to election of non-European members. This will hopefully enable ESPE to improve further, increase the number and quality of its members and eventually become a real worldwide Society for Paediatric Endocrinology.'[191]

After a heated discussion, the members then decided by a majority to delete the term 'exceptionally' in article 2 of the constitution. Two further proposed changes to the constitution – both in article 6 – which should remove existing obstacles to applications, were discussed controversially. One suggestion was to remove the requirement that an applicant should have presented an abstract or paper at an Annual Meeting, but need only to express an active interest and knowledge in the field of paediatric endocrinology. It was also proposed that candidates should have to submit only one letter of recommendation, and not, as previously required, two. However neither amendment achieved the necessary two-thirds majority, and the old criteria for candidature remained in force.[192]

187   Minutes of Annual Business Meeting, 2001.
188   Minutes of Annual Business Meeting, 2001.
189   Minutes of Annual Business Meeting, 2002.
190   Secretary's Annual Report, 2005.
191   Secretary's Annual Report, 2005.
192   Minutes of Annual Business Meeting, 2005.

ESPE Becomes a Global Organisation

Membership and Annual Meetings

Following ESPE's initial opening up to non-European candidates in 2001 and 2005, expansion in subsequent years was pursued more boldly. In February 2006, Ze'ev Hochberg proposed creating an additional membership category specially for members from third world countries. They should be exempt from membership fees but still be eligible to vote.[193] The aim was to attract new members and further raise ESPE's international profile.

In 2009, 74 candidates applied for membership and were accepted by Council. 28 of them were from countries outside Europe, 10 came from South Korea. ESPE thus counted 677 members. The internationalisation of the organisation was to be promoted further on various levels. In the same year Ze'ev Hochberg suggested that the Council should aim to include a member from a non-European country in its ranks.[194]

In 2010 'a respectable number of 66 applications' were received.[195] The Secretary's Annual Report stated:

'This high number was largely attributed to the newly simplified eligibility criteria and promoting ESPE membership throughout the world. I would like to point out that in 2004 a mere 21 applications were received. This represents, therefore, a huge success and means that we are working in the right direction to make ESPE a true international society. In fact many new members are from outside Europe and the Mediterranean countries. We must all strive to do our best to continue to invest in improving education and research and strengthen ESPE leadership in Paediatric Endocrinology and Diabetes around the world.'[196]

The Annual Meetings also became increasingly more international. The 45th Annual Meeting in Rotterdam in 2006 was attended by 1,823 delegates, 322 from non-European countries.[197]

At the 46th ESPE Annual Meeting in Helsinki there were '2,104 delegates from 87 countries, compared with 71 countries in the previous year'.[198]

The Annual Meeting in 2008, which was held in Istanbul, was 'the first time that an annual conference has been organized in a city that has a 'foothold' in both Europe and Asia'.[199] Speakers had been invited from Asia, China and India.

---

193 Minutes of Council Meeting, 18th–19th February 2006, Rome.
194 Minutes of Annual Business Meeting; Secretary's Annual Report, 2009.
195 Secretary's Annual Report, 2010.
196 Secretary's Annual Report, 2010.
197 Secretary's Annual Report, 2007.
198 Secretary's Annual Report, 2008.
199 ESPE Newsletter, Summer 2008, Issue 9.

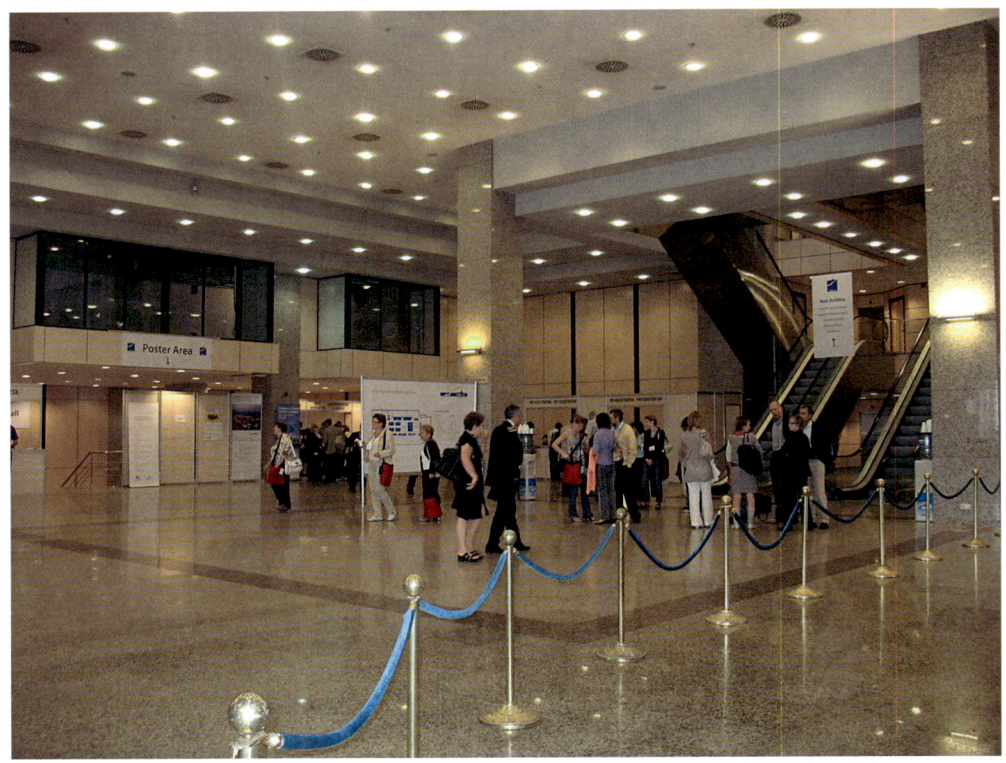

Insights into the modern congress building of the Annual Meeting in Istanbul, 2008.

This meeting was important as having been designed by its President, Atilla Büyükgebiz, as 'an environmentally friendly event'[200] – printed material should be used as little as possible. ESPE is committed to make a contribution to environmental protection. In order to document the environmental awareness of ESPE and 'in celebration of ESPE's European origins'[201] an 'ESPE 2008 Memorial Forest' was created in 2008, sponsored by Novo Nordisk Turkey. It is located on Mount Izmir, 450 km from Istanbul, and should 'act as a symbol of the Society's "growing" future'. 3,000 trees were planted. Every delegate at that year's meeting had a tree planted and received a certificate in commemoration of this historic event.[202]

In 2009, the Annual Meeting was the 8th LWPES/ESPE Joint Meeting, held from 9th–12th September in New York, with Paul Saenger and Francesco Chiarelli as presidents. It was attended by more than 3,600 delegates, the largest number ever at a

---

200 ESPE Newsletter, Summer 2008, Issue 9.
201 ESPE Newsletter, Summer 2008, Issue 9.
202 ESPE Newsletter, Summer 2008, Issue 9.

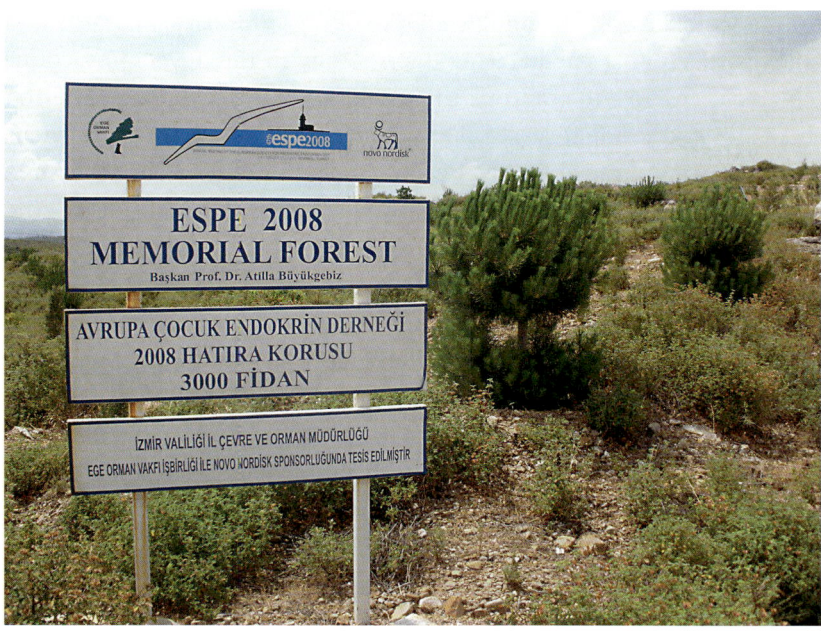

The ESPE Memorial Forest, 2008. 3,000 trees were planted as a symbol of the Society's 'growing' future.

Joint Meeting. The Annual Meeting in Prague in 2010 was also extremely successful. During the Business Meeting Franco Chiarelli expressed his thanks 'for an excellent meeting in Prague and reported that it was the biggest ever ESPE meeting, with almost 3,000 delegates from 91 countries'.[203] 700 delegates came from countries outside Europe.[204]

Paediatric Endocrinology in Developing Countries[205]

ESPE's advancement to a global organisation is also reflected in the development of new teaching and training programmes. Courses and projects have been organised in Africa, India and China, and a training centre has been established in Nairobi, where the idea of on-going training in a developing country in the subspecialty paediatric endocrinology has been very successfully realised.

203   Minutes Annual Business Meeting, 2010.
204   Minutes Annual Business Meeting, 2010.
205   For the new education programs see the ESPE Website: http://eurospe.org/education/education_developing-countries.html; http://eurospe.org/education/education_maghrebProject.html.

Leading World-Wide

The programme 'Paediatric Endocrinology in Developing Countries' was launched in 2004. The goal was to support paediatric endocrinology in the developing countries, and particularly in Africa, to improve the medical care of children suffering from diabetes and other endocrine diseases. This should be achieved through teaching programmes, visits by young scientists to Europe, the free supply of journals such as *Hormone Research* and, finally, through the establishment of a training centre. ESPE pledged financial support amounting to EUR 50.000, which was covered partly by UNICEF Italy and Novo Nordisk Italy.[206]

The first teaching programme was run with the support of Professor Angela Okolo from October 14th–17th, 2005 at the University of Benin in Nigeria,[207] where Cecilia Camacho-Hübner, John Gregory, Marc Maes, Otto Westphal and Martin Ritzén held an introductory course for young Nigerian paediatricians. This course was structured on similar lines to the Winter School. The 21 students, 8 men and 13 women, were aged between 30 and 45 and came from 18 different Nigerian universities.

Martin Ritzén reported on this first course: 'We were impressed by the high level of textbook knowledge, but surprised to find that less attention was being paid to important aspects of patient work-up, such as taking a detailed history and performing and interpreting a careful physical examination. Less than half of the students, all specialists in paediatrics, were using growth charts in their clinical work!'[208] The course was successful, and a second, similar course was held from 16th to 20th May 2006 in Nairobi, Kenya.

The Nairobi Training Centre
The Nairobi Training Centre was launched in May 2008 with the 'Programme for Fellowship on Paediatric Endocrinology and Diabetes in Africa'. The training programme was coordinated and organised from a private, non-profit-making hospital, the Gertrude Children's Hospital. Two other large hospitals, the Aga Khan and the Kenyatta, were also involved. This programme is sponsored primarily by the World Diabetes Foundation (WDF) and supported by ESPE.

The eight scholars came from Nigeria, Tanzania and Kenya. The course lasted 15 months and included clinic consultations, ward rounds, lectures by tutors, seminars, journal club presentations and many discussions between the fellows and tutors. ESPE members served as tutors for a month at a time.

---

206 Secretary's Annual Report, 2005.
207 M. Ritzén, Report following the first Africa course: ESPE Course on Paediatric Endocrinology at the University of Benin, 4th–17th October, 2005.
208 M. Ritzén, Report following the first Africa course: ESPE Course on Paediatric Endocrinology at the University of Benin, 4th–17th October, 2005.

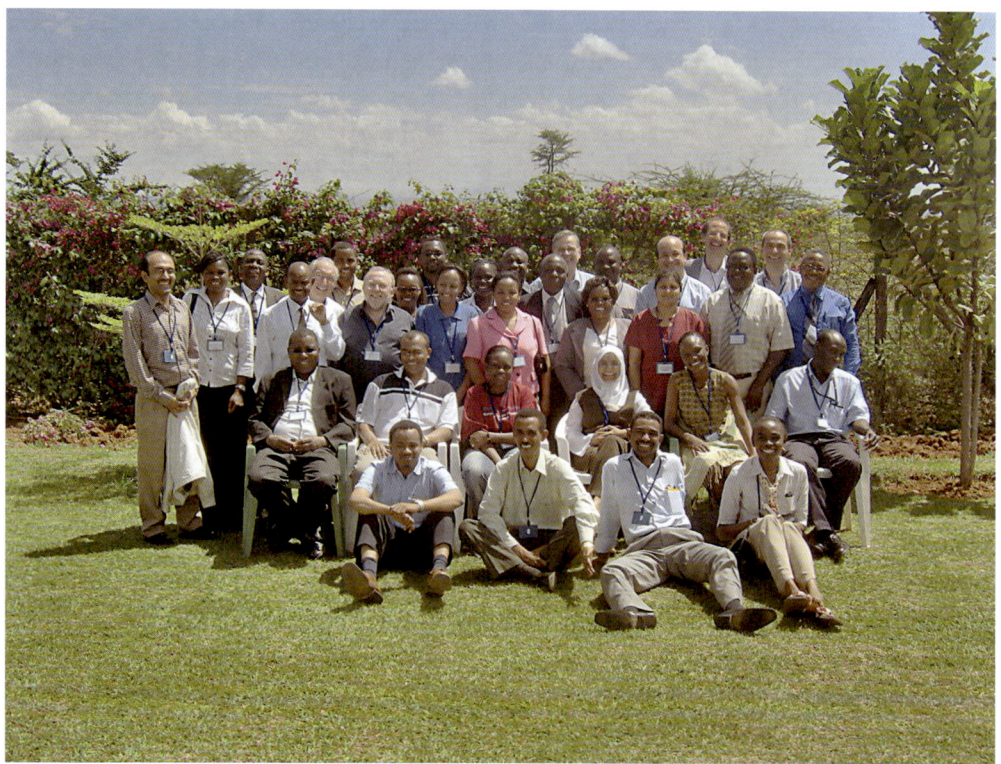

Participants of the successful teaching programme in Nairobi (Kenya), May 2006.

ESPE Maghreb Project

Given the success of the ESPE Africa project based in Kenya and the clear need for ESPE input in the francophone Maghreb countries, planning began on a further project. The aim of the ESPE Maghreb Project is to improve the training of paediatricians in the French speaking countries of North Africa. It is planned to hold meetings once a year lasting five days, with European and North African lecturers and 25 students who will be selected by the two committees, the North Africa Committee and the ESPE Maghreb School Steering Committee. Both lecturers and students should present cases and research projects for general discussion. The programme is being financed, initially for three years, by Pfizer. The first 'Maghreb School in French of the European Society for Paediatric Endocrinology' will be held in Casablanca, Morocco, from 21st to 27th October 2011.

China and India

In 2007 ESPE approached the Chinese Society for Paediatric Endocrinology and Metabolism (CSPEM) with the aim of supporting paediatric endocrinology in China. In collaboration with the Chinese colleagues it was decided to run a course for young paediatricians that was similar to the Summer School. The first Chinese Fellows'

Course, in which 2 ESPE members and 5 Chinese lecturers taught 27 participants, was held from November 3rd to 4th, 2009 in Yangzhou, about 300 kilometres north of Shanghai.[209]

ESPE also forged contacts with India. The first Paediatric Endocrinology Training Programme of the ISPAE (Indian Society for Paediatric and Adolescent Endocrinology) was held in New Delhi from November 10th to 13th, 2009. It was organised with ESPE support by the ISPAE and the Indian Academy of Paediatrics 'for the benefit of students and young faculty'.[210] As in China the main structure was largely inspired by the ESPE Summer School, with a mix of small group sessions, plenary lectures and plenary case presentations. In his Annual Report in 2010, Secretary Francesco Chiarelli wrote: 'Altogether, we consider that the interaction with the Indian group has been excellent and very beneficial to all and should be encouraged in the future: in particular, Indian faculty and more senior fellows will be encouraged to come to the ESPE meeting [...].'[211]

Global Paediatric Endocrinology and Diabetes
Global Paediatric Endocrinology and Diabetes (GPED), which was founded in 2010, is an international forum whose goal is 'to improve the care of children in developing countries with endocrine disorders through the provision of training and educational opportunities, developing research studies and promoting advocacy for our goals'. All national paediatric endocrine societies are represented and it is chaired by Ze'ev Hochberg. There are currently 56 active members, of whom 14 are also ESPE members.[212]

Annual Meetings and Scientific Contributions – 'Number Versus Quality'?

In 2006 under item 6 of the agenda – 'Number versus quality' – the quality of posters presented at the Annual Meetings was discussed at the Council Meeting in Rome.[213] This question had been debated repeatedly within the Society since the late 1970s following the introduction of posters at the first Rotterdam meeting in 1976. After lengthy deliberations the POC decided that all submitted posters should be shown in future. Congrex would be responsible for ensuring there was sufficient exhibition space.[214]

On the one hand, the ever-increasing number of poster sessions organised in this way led to a diversity of quality and topics, and benefited the not so well established younger colleagues.

209 Minutes of Annual Business Meeting, 2010.
210 Secretary's Annual Report, 2010.
211 Secretary's Annual Report, 2010.
212 Secretary's Annual Report, 2010.
213 Minutes of Council Meeting, 18th–19th February 2006, Rome.
214 Minutes of Council Meeting, 30th June 2006, Rotterdam.

On the other hand, it was important that visitors should be able to rely on the quality of the research presented.

Quality Assurance and New Awards

In the new millennium, with the opening up of ESPE and the Annual Meetings, a systematic selection and ranking of the submitted scientific contributions is indispensable. In order to improve the quality of abstracts, the POC decided in 2006 to experimentally 're-introduce the scheme whereby each abstract submitted for the Annual Meeting had to be sponsored by an ESPE member' who should review the abstract in question. It was agreed, however, that the sponsoring rule should not be applied too strictly, so that unsponsored abstracts could also be accepted.[215] There is still a strict peer-review process: in 2006 5% of all submitted abstracts were not accepted, but 'read by title' only. A stricter ruling was decided on for 2007, where 10% of the submissions were 'read by title'.[216] For the meeting in Istanbul in 2008, with 180 positions to be filled, ESPE members were given the opportunity to act as reviewers.[217]

In addition to the established mechanisms for selecting abstracts and abstract rankings, competitions and awards play an important role in quality assurance. The recognition of particularly high-quality contributions can create incentives for further excellence while at the same time, regardless of the diversity and heterogeneity of the scientific content presented, imparting a binding standard of scientific quality. Since the Annual Meeting in Helsinki in 2007, the *ESPE President's Poster Award* is presented to the five best posters shown at an Annual Meeting. The winners receive an official ESPE award diploma and a present from the President, and are included in the official list of ESPE award winners.[218]

The '*Hormone Research in Paediatrics Prize*', endowed with EUR 4,000, has been awarded by Karger Publishers since 2004 in order to encourage the submission of top research manuscripts from young scientists. It is presented during the Annual Meeting with the other ESPE awards in the fields of clinical and experimental research for the 'best original, peer reviewed paper published in HRP in the field of Paediatric Endocrinology in the last 12 months'.[219]

Since 2004, clinical focus sessions – 'symposia-type sessions composed of delegates abstract submissions'[220] – are held during the Annual Meeting. Only the best

---

215 Minutes of Council Meeting, 16th May 2005, Brussels; Minutes of Council Meeting, 18th–19th February 2006, Rome.
216 Minutes of Council Meeting, 30th June 2006, Rotterdam.
217 Minutes of Council Meeting, 17th–18th February 2007, Rome.
218 Minutes of Council Meeting, 30th June 2006, Rotterdam; ESPE Homepage.
219 Minutes of Council Meeting, 24th January 2004, London.
220 Minutes of Program Organising Committee, 2004.

abstracts are presented so the ESPE Programme Organising Committee has decided to limit the number of presentations per session to three or two contributions.[221]

Training Meets 'Top Science'

Since 2008, pursuing different objectives than with most of its other activities, ESPE has organised several conferences under the heading Recent Progress in Paediatric Endocrinology (RPPE): 'unlike the other ESPE projects which are aimed at trainees, the RPPE is aimed at placing ESPE at the top scientific world'.[222]

The first conference, The Nobel Conference on System Biology & Child Health, was supported by the Nobel Foundation and held in May 2008 in Stockholm, to bring world class scientists and paediatric endocrinologists together to consider how top science can be better used to help children with endocrine disorders. In 2009, the series was renamed New Inroads in Child Health (NICHe).

The aim of the newly established *ESPE Science School* is to put young paediatricians in touch with top science, covering the fields of statistics, epidemiology, molecular and systems biology, and methods in writing and presenting science. This programme is supported by Pfizer. The first ESS was held in Varberg, Sweden from May 23rd to 26th, 2010, and was attended by 20 students and 12 teachers. The students were final year PhD students, postdoctoral fellows and young faculty members with a special interest in paediatric endocrinology. The teachers were ESPE members and speakers who had been at the NICHe Conference.[223]

In conclusion, ESPE started as a small club of scientists in the new medical field of paediatric endocrinology in 1962. This club developed into a society and this field of work, which now also included paediatric and adolescent diabetology, became an officially recognised medical subspecialty. As paediatric endocrinology grew and embraced new topics, so did ESPE. As the number of prizes, training programmes and fellowships increased, ESPE became 'a truly global Society with members from the USA, the Middle East, Australia, South America and the Far East'.[224]

Looking back on ESPE's impressive growth and development during its infancy, childhood, adolescence, early and middle adulthood, we can now, on its 50th anniversary, feel extremely confident about its future in the years to come.

For further details on ESPE's latest developments and activities, please see the ESPE Homepage at www.eurospe.org.

221 Minutes of Program Organising Committee, 2004.
222 Minutes of Council Meeting, 17th–18th February 2007, Rome.
223 Secretary's Annual Report, 2010.
224 Pers. Recoll., Martin Savage, pp. 111–114 in this book.

Personal Recollections

ESPE
50

ESPE Is in Good Health

Jesús Argente, Spain

I first heard about the European Society for Paediatric Endocrinology (ESPE) during my training in paediatrics (1981–1984) in Madrid, Spain, and then in paediatric endocrinology (1984–1986) in Paris, France. My mentor in Paris, Professor Jean-Claude Job, as well as my mentor in Spain, Professor Manuel Hernández, invited me to present some abstracts at the 25th ESPE Annual meeting in Zurich and also at the next meeting in Toulouse.

I cannot forget these meetings because I had the opportunity to meet the people responsible for the development of paediatric endocrinology in Europe, including Professor Andrea Prader, Ruth Illig, Milo Zachmann, Zvi Laron, among others. I was very impressed with the scientific atmosphere and very pleased at having the possibility to speak in a very open manner to these people that I only knew by name.

I still remember my flight from Zurich to Paris talking to Professor Job about the importance of the scientific method to be applied to our patients in order to conduct clinical research and to make progress in our understanding of the pathophysiology of human diseases. As a very young doctor starting his academic career in paediatric endocrinology, I was very eager about having this opportunity to learn and advance my training in this field.

I became an ESPE member in 1988 with the generous support of Professor Job. Since 1989 I have attended all ESPE meetings. I have had the opportunity to present 120 scientific abstracts during this time, interacting with colleagues in Paediatric Endocrinology around the world. In addition, I am in debt to ESPE for having awarded me the Henning Andersen Prize during the Annual Meeting in Vienna in 1990. It was also very important for my career to obtain the ESPE Young Investigator Award during the Joint LWPES/ESPE Meeting in San Francisco in 1993. A very special and memorable moment occurred when I had the opportunity to become ESPE President and organize the 41st ESPE Annual Meeting in Madrid, Spain. It was during this meeting that the new ESPE logo was first used.

ESPE has represented friendship, advancement in scientific knowledge, human and scientific relationships, personal progress, consolidation of my own paediatric endocrinology group, opportunities for a great number of fellows in my group and laboratory to have their first contact with a scientific meeting and the first possibility to communicate their own scientific findings. ESPE has allowed me the opportunity to send Fellows abroad who today are independent researchers (Luis Pérez-Jurado, Silvia González-Parra, José Carlos Moreno, among others), as well as to receive foreign Fellows in my group (special mention to my Brazilian Fellows).

It has been, and is still, a great pleasure to have the opportunity to serve as editor of the ESPE Newsletter. This was an excellent idea to keep ESPE members in touch with what our society is doing.

My participation as member and Chairman of the Scientific Committee for Short and Long-term ESPE Fellowships has been a marvellous experience, giving me the possibility to interact with many colleagues and also to develop friendships. Special thanks in this regard to my friends Wieland Kiess, Michel Polak, Leo Dunkel and Anders Juul.

In the ESPE's 50th anniversary year, we are proud to know that it has become the most important scientific society for paediatric endocrinology in the world. Hence, ESPE is in good health; however, one of ESPE's challenges is to maintain this quality in the future. Therefore, all ESPE members, including the new members and especially the younger people, will need to continue working hard to develop good scientific groups and good science. Everyone must make an extra effort so that ESPE can maintain its leadership.

Some Milestones in the Development of Paediatric Endocrinology in Belgium and ESPE

Jean-Pierre Bourguignon and Marc Maes, Belgium, on behalf of the Belgian Study Group for Paediatric Endocrinology (BSGPE)

During the past 50 years, paediatric endocrinology went through a dramatic expansion in many aspects: the increased core of knowledge, the number of scientific publications, the growth-promoting therapies, etc. Throughout that process, the global paediatric perspective has fortunately been retained with the whole patient as the main focus. In addition, self-criticism has been crucial for temperance of enthusiasm resulting from exponential increase of possibilities in patient management and research.

The aim of this contribution is to give some examples of advances and self-critical attitudes over the past 40 years that have been central to the development of paediatric endocrinology in Belgium and in ESPE through Belgian delegates. Three periods will be considered.

The 1980s, Belgian Pioneers in Paediatric Endocrinology
A group was convened by the Belgian public authorities in 1974 to create a committee for treatment of pituitary dwarfism. All were paediatric endocrinologists except for Marc Vandeweghe who was an internist. Among the early BSGPE members in the 1970s, Rita Craen, Marc Du Caju, Christian Ernould and Paul Malvaux have retired. Renée Wolter and Marc Vandeweghe have passed away and Guy Van Vliet has moved to Montreal.

A first lesson drawn from those days of limited biological imaging and genetic assessments was the paramount importance of thorough clinical evaluation. This is still true despite the giant progress made by molecular studies. A second lesson came from exposure to a peer review process. Though our mentors were outstanding paediatric endocrinologists, they were eager to put individual practice into question and

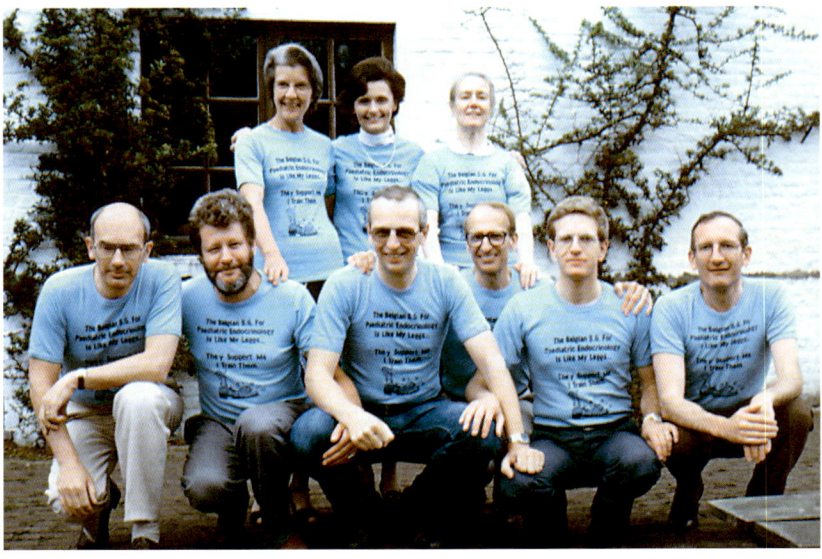

From left to right: Renée Wolter, Magda Lodeweyckx, Rita Craen (upper row); Christian Ernould, Marc Vandeweghe, Jean-Pierre Bourguignon, Paul Malvaux, Guy Van Vliet, Marc Du Caju.

benefit from colleagues' comments. We have been privileged in sharing the excellence in clinical tradition and revision of attitudes with our pioneering colleagues. Such a peer review process at monthly national meetings has been maintained since then and is felt to be a precious heritage from our mentors.

Among the early Belgian scientific contributions, Renée Wolter added to the rationale of a neonatal screening for congenital hypothyroidism by demonstrating loss of IQ in relation to postnatal delay in initiating thyroxine substitution [1]. The late François Delange provided evidence of iodine deficiency throughout the world, including Europe where deficiency was almost silent but definitely needed correction [2]. Therapeutic education of patients and families facing type-1-diabetes is a difficult condition where compliance was questioned and assistance provided by educating nurses at home and at school [3].

The 1990s, Childhood of Paediatric Endocrinology in Belgium
A priming of further self-criticism of our management of paediatric endocrine patients arose from collaborative Belgian studies with psychologists. In girls treated for sexual precocity, the concern of paediatric endocrinologists about adult height was expected while the patient distress from early breast development could be underestimated [4]. In Turner girls, it appeared that short stature perception and the consequent justification of GH treatment were rather weak before 5–6 years of age [5]. This led us to balance the final height benefits of early GH therapy against acceptability in very young patients.

Self-criticism also belongs to teaching experiences as long as we allow the trainees to put ourselves into question. This was true during an ESPE training initiative, the 1st ESPE Winter School in Hungary in 1996 that was chaired by Ze'ev Hochberg. He was concerned by the bias linked to infallibility of ESPE teachers as viewed by the attendees, a possible prejudice to the development of self-criticism. Thus, the ESPE teachers including JP Bourguignon were asked by Ze'ev to start with a clinical case where they failed. It worked so well that it resulted in some kind of mini-revolution, and long debriefing with the participants was needed.

In 1999, the 5th International Conference on the Control of the Onset of Puberty was held in Liège [6]. Since Belgium had a long-standing tradition of cartoons and comics, we took this opportunity to have Franx, a Belgian caricaturist, immortalize some participants who are shown in the portrait gallery on pp. 68–69.

The 2000s, Adolescence of Paediatric Endocrinology in Belgium

2000 was the year when the 39th Annual Meeting of ESPE took place in Brussels. This was a collaborative challenge for the members of the BSGPE to participate in the organization of the Meeting and to contribute to its success. As stated in the Presidential welcome address by Marc Maes, the Meeting was a unique opportunity for us to celebrate Paul Malvaux's retirement. Paul was one of the 3 musketeers who gave birth to paediatric endocrinology in Belgium. Paul was himself a former President of the early ESPE Meeting held in Leuven. One of Paul's anecdotes was the telephone call from A. Bongiovanni, one of the pioneer figures of paediatric endocrinology in the US, asking him whether there was a connecting flight between Brussels and Leuven, not knowing that the two cities were 20 km apart! At that time only 200 paediatricians participated in the Meeting sharing commodities in the University Dorms.

The 2000 Meeting saw new initiatives such as the mini-programme at a glance, still used nowadays, such as representative booths of our Society and Karger Publishers during our Meetings, and interactive voting sessions stimulating the interaction between participants and the speaker.

Future

The BSGPE is facing new challenges. The steady increase in the numbers of members affiliated to the BSGPE has increased the workload of our monthly meetings, requiring a new organization. Also new working groups centred on specific themes such as sexual differentiation, obesity and, in the near future, diabetes were recently created. The new BSGPE consists now of 32 members, where peer review still takes place and we still ask each other advice about difficult medical situations, where study protocols are discussed and commented, and where the interest of individual centres is still balanced against the interest of the group. New members have joined the BSGPE and will certainly contribute to the bright future of the BSGPE – and surely join ESPE and contribute to that too.

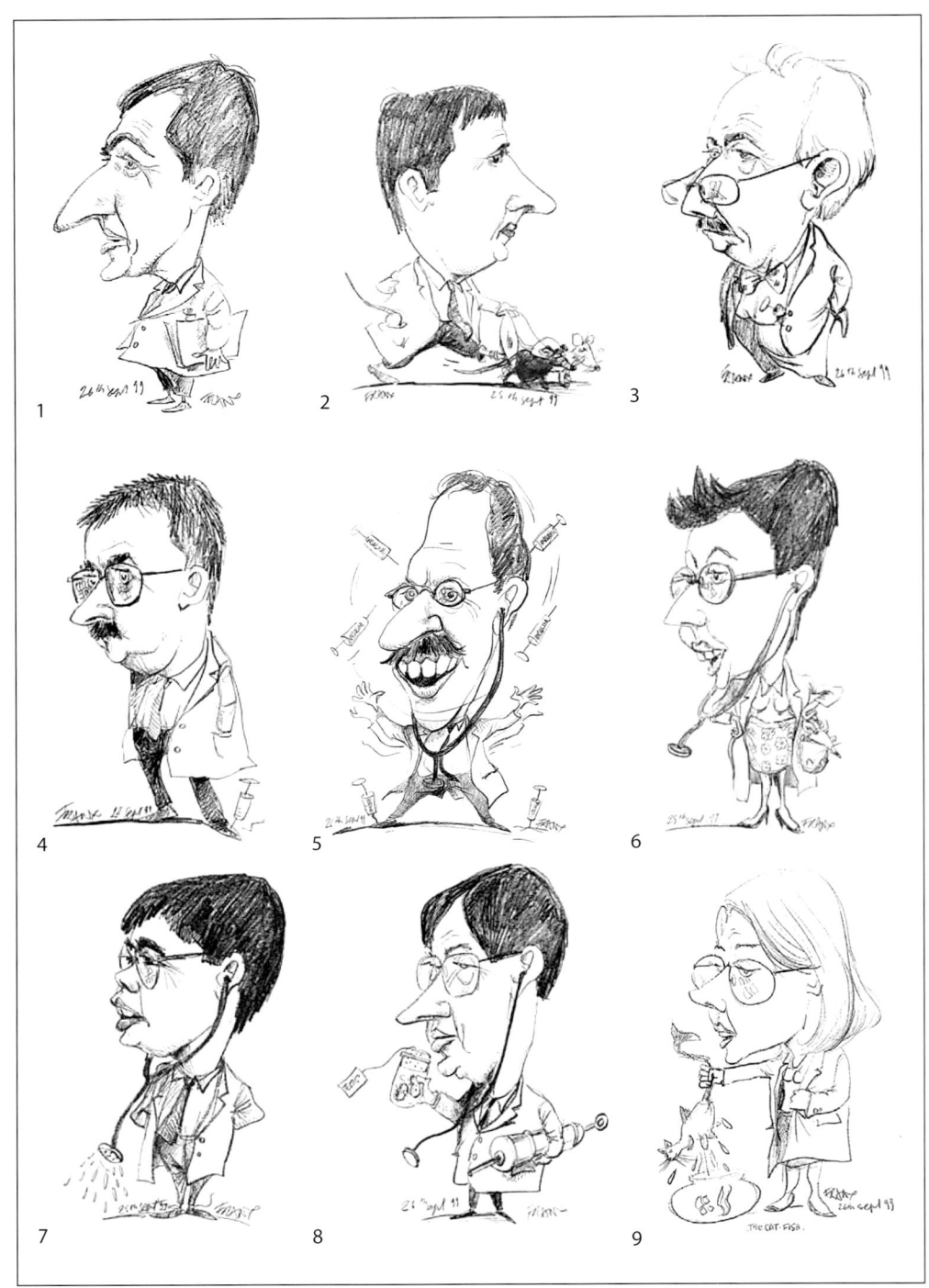

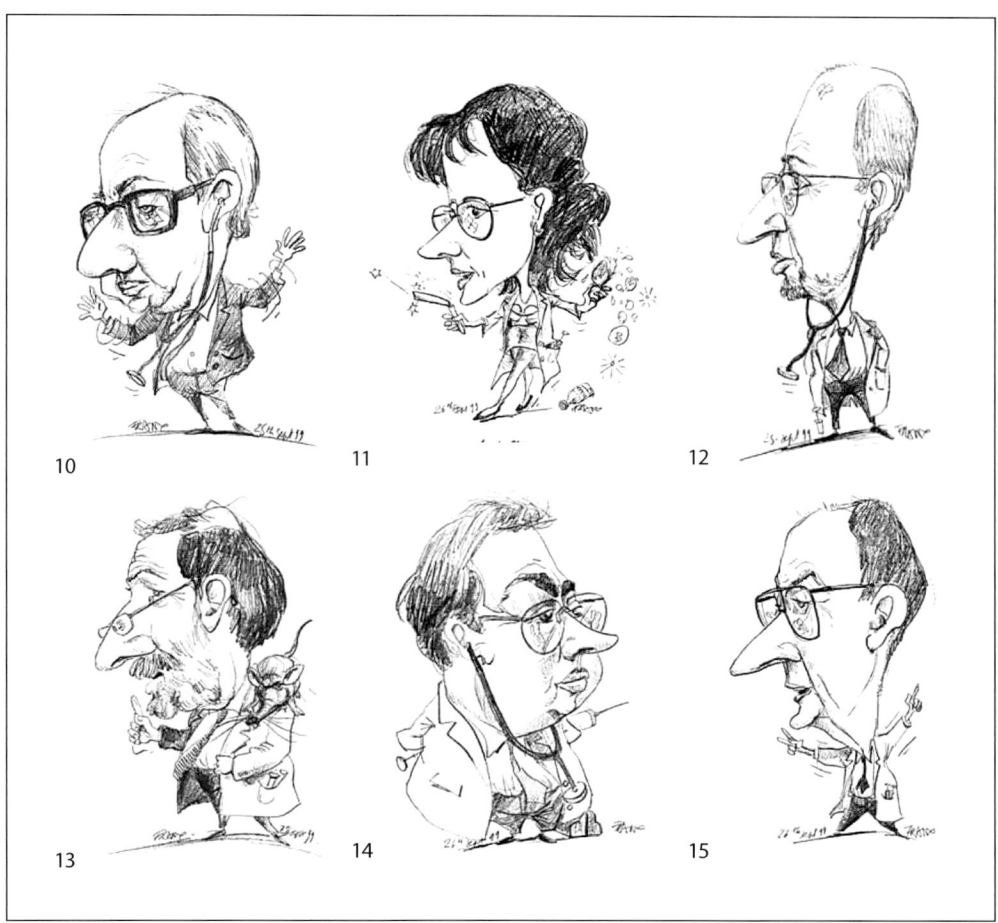

Franx, a Belgian caricaturist, immortalized some participants who are shown in the portrait gallery. Can you guess who is who? See p. 70 for the answers. Adapted from Bourguignon and Plant [6], with permission of the publisher and the caricatured scientists.

References

1 Wolter R, Noël P, De Cock P, Craen M, Ernould C, Malvaux P, Verstaeten F, Simons J, Mertens S, Van Broeck N, Vanderschueren-Lodeweyckx M: Neuropsychological study in treated thyroid dysgenesis. Acta Paediatr Scand 1979;(suppl 227):41–46.

2 Delange F, Heidemann P, Bourdoux P, Larsson A, Vigneri R, Klett M, Beckers C, Stubbe P: Regional variations of iodine nutrition and thyroid function during the neonatal period in Europe. Biol Neonate 1986;49:322–330.

3 Ernould C, Bourguignon JP, Vanderschueren-Lodeweyckx M, Wolter R, Malvaux P, Craen M, Du Caju MV, Franchimont P : Hypopituitarism and idiopathic delayed puberty: a longitudinal study in an attempt to diagnose gonadotropin deficiency before puberty. Pediatr Adolesc Endocr 1982;10:43–46.

4 Xhrouet-Heinrichs D, Lagrou K, Heinrichs C, Craen M, Dooms L, Malvaux P, Kanen F, Bourguignon JP: Longitudinal study of behavioral and affective patterns in girls with central precocious puberty during long-acting triptorelin therapy. Acta Paediatrica 1997;86:808–815.

5 Lagrou K, Xhrouet-Heinrichs D, Heinrichs C, Craen M, Chanoine JP, Malvaux P, Bourguignon JP: Age-related perception of stature, acceptance of therapy, and psychosocial functioning in human growth hormone-treated girls with Turner's syndrome. J Clin Endocrinol Metab 1998;83:1494–1501.

6 Bourguignon JP, Plant T (eds): The Onset of Puberty in Perspective. Excerpta Medica International Congress Series, 1202. Amsterdam, Elsevier, 2000.

Solution to figure on pp. 68–69: 1 = Raimo Voutilainen; 2 = Richard Stanhope; 3 = Pierre Sizonenko; 4 = Peter Clayton; 5 = Roelof Odink; 6 = Henriette Delemarre; 7 = Fred Wu; 8 = Niels Erik Skakkebaek; 9 = Heike Jung; 10 = Martin Savage; 11 = Lourdes Ibanez; 12 = Jean-Pierre Bourguignon; 13 = Michel Aubert; 14 = Charles Sultan; 15 = Ieuan Hughes.

We Were Young and Very Enthusiastic

Giuseppe Chiumello, Italy

In 1965, Professor Andrea Prader contacted my Professor to know whether anyone who was involved in endocrinology was interested in participating in the European Society for Paediatric Endocrinology meeting organized by Professor William Hamilton, which was to be held in Glasgow in 1966. From that day on an amazing adventure started. On that occasion I met the pioneers of paediatric endocrinology: Illig, Rappaport, Tanner, Aarskog, Laron, Francois, Bertrand. I was immediately stunned by the young age of the participants, their liveliness during discussions, and the sympathy that was shared among all. Furthermore, the Annual Meeting was looked forward to with great excitement and also trepidation.

In 1980, I had the privilege of organising the Annual Meeting in Bergamo, historical city of Northern Italy. Everything had been arranged by the hospital personnel. No travel agency was used and sponsors were scarce. The speakers were accommodated in the Archbishop's Seminary in Bergamo Alta: a very evocative setting although uncomfortable to some (some colleagues complained and a taxi service had to be organized to transfer guests from the lower city to the congress site). I will not speak about the scientific program in detail, but I remember the high academic level and the participation of certain American colleagues: Baxter, New, Drash, Becker.

The social programme was extraordinary. The weather was wonderful and the sky was always blue in the magnificent medieval city. A memorable vocal concert took place in the Basilica of Santa Maria Maggiore: an unforgettable setting and chorus who interpreted music from the Italian Renaissance. The most extraordinary event was the dinner which took place in the Malpaga Castle, built in the 16th century, during which improvised dances were performed to the music interpreted by the barber of the village who played the accordion.

Do not misjudge me if I only spoke about the social aspects of the event: we were young and very enthusiastic. The majority of us paid their own travel expenses and accommodation. Sponsoring agencies were few and everything weighed on our salary and the meagre financial credit of our institution.

Personal Recollections

Souvenirs of ESPE : I Remember

Paul Czernichow, France

I remember when ESPE was a small group of paediatricians fascinated by the development of new science in endocrinology. This group came from all over Europe which, in a sense, was an example of what Europe could achieve when working together on a specific project. In some ways, this pre-empted what Europe would be in the future and what it is now.

I went to my first ESPE meeting in 1969 (Malmö, Sweden) when recently qualified in paediatrics but still studying paediatric endocrinology. I was inexperienced and much impressed by the scientific presentations of specialists from major European centres.

I remember the passionate spirit for learning, friendship, scientific rigour and open discussions. I don't remember any spirit of competition, nor conflicts or aggression (though it was probably present) but I do remember open exchange, a desire to learn, to compare experiences and build a new corpus of knowledge based on the most recent advances of science.

I remember that in 1974 my mentor Professor Pierre Royer was the ESPE president and organized the Annual Meeting in Paris. The number of participants was probably no more than 200. At that time, we felt that it was possible to arrange a social gathering and invite colleagues into our homes to have dinner together. We organized ourselves into 10 groups and I remember a memorable evening when I welcomed 20 colleagues at my home. Many of them are still ESPE members and friends. Can you imagine doing such a thing today? Just impossible. ESPE is now a large and well-established society of doctors coming from all over Europe and the world which, inevitably, has lost some of the charm and intimacy of a small community.

I remember when the first ESPE Summer School took place. With a group of colleagues we decided to launch a new ESPE 'product': a 2–3 days' seminar with the ambition of a high level teaching for a small group of very motivated ESPE 'students', all young paediatricians in their 30s still engaged in paediatric endocrinology

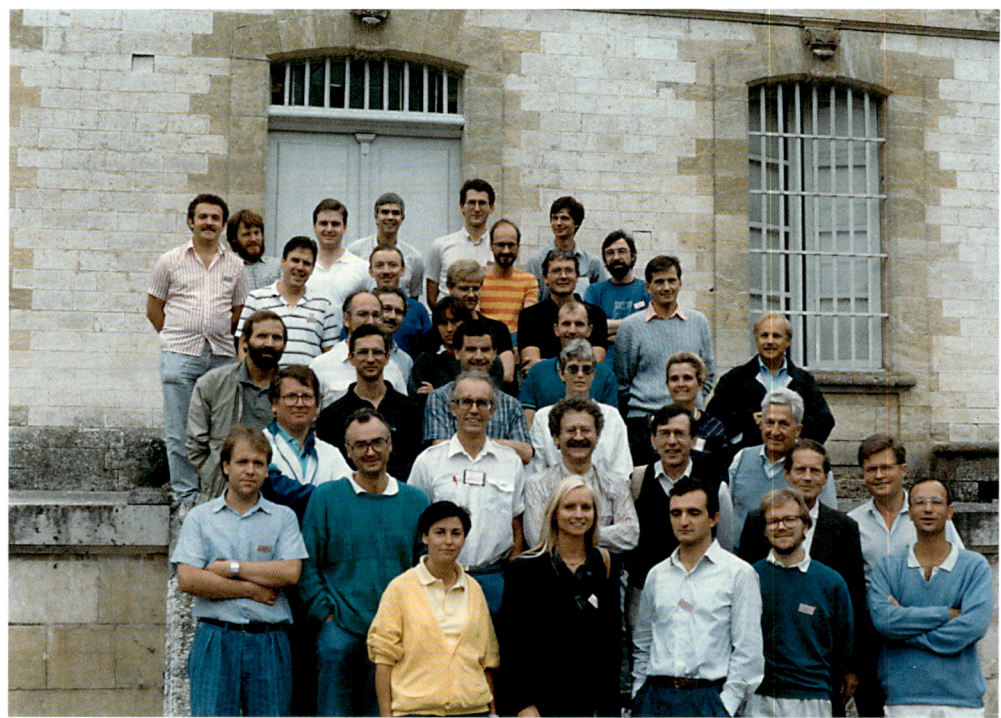

Participants of the first ESPE Summer School in 1987. We were having a good time indeed! Paul Czernichow is in the middle second row between Martin Ritzén and Leo Van den Brande. You may see Alfred Jost with white curly hair to the right of Leo. Just behind Paul you see Kerstin Albertsson-Wikland and behind her Ieuan Hughes. Behind Alfred Jost you may see Pierre Sizonenko. Try to guess who these young students are now and where they are. Most of them now have key positions in their universities.

training. Our objective was to identify and 'recruit' those paediatric endocrinologists who were likely to become the future teachers and leaders in the field. This is exactly what happened. Leo Van den Brande was very supportive and helped me to establish the ground rules which, by the way, are still in use today. We set up a scientific committee responsible for choosing the topics and inviting the teachers. Teaching was undertaken by ESPE members but also by scientists from outside our community. And a process for selecting students was established. To reduce the cost, it was decided to plan the Summer School just before or after the annual ESPE meeting. It was the responsibility of the ESPE President to make all practical arrangements. The venue was to be close to where the Annual Meeting was held, in informal surroundings, to encourage interaction between students and teachers. An important issue was the financial aspect of this enterprise. The ESPE budget was very small then and it was not possible to finance this event from our own resources. I was fortunate at that time to work with Ferring on the use of DDAVP in children and to work closely with Frederik Paulsen, a man of vision and ethics. So I asked him if he would support this project; his answer was enthusiastic and positive. Yes, he said, I will support this for 3 years, and then we will evaluate the impact. After 3 years, he decided to continue and, as you know, Ferring is still our ESPE Summer School sponsor. Thank you, Frederik.

I remember that the first venue was in France. Pierre Rochiccioli was President and the Summer School was held in Chateau Bonas, a small city south west of Toulouse; a charming little castle, in the middle of the country. We were lucky to have a group of renowned teachers: Alfred Jost taught sex development, giving a historical perspective and looking at the most recent developments; we invited Inder Verma, a US scientist from San Diego who talked about oncogenes - and many other teachers, members of the ESPE. I remember too with pleasure the students, many of whom have now top responsibilities at their respective universities! Obviously we made good choices.

I remember that the atmosphere of the scientific presentations was less formal than now, though with the same scientific rigour. I was in Ulm for the Annual ESPE meeting in 1979 where I was proud to have a paper accepted for an oral presentation. This was the result of a collaborative research with a German colleague on the presence of circulating anti-vasopressin cell antibodies in the serum of patients with diabetes insipidus. This colleague and I were quite disorganized; I was sure that since he was the first author, he would present the paper – and he was certain that I would be the speaker! The session was chaired by Selna Kaplan and Bob Blizzard, the latter being my mentor when I was a fellow at Johns Hopkins' Hospital in Baltimore. When my turn came, my German colleague was asked to present but he was not in the room – he was not even in town! Remember that in those days, we were using the old-fashion slides to present. So Bob Blizzard announced: Paul, you are the author of this paper; you should know your data! I will call the next speaker and you have 15 minutes to prepare your talk! We were in a university amphitheatre with all the facilities - meaning blackboard and chalk. Those 15 minutes were one of the most intense periods of my life. I was not an experienced speaker and this was quite a challenge. Finally I presented my work talking and writing on the blackboard, answering questions with the data always visible on the board. I remember that the audience was very appreciative but I was exhausted! This is an example of how relaxed and informal the scientific presentations could be at that time.

I have no nostalgia of this period. ESPE now is just different in style. I think that it remains a unique place for scientific excellence, exchange and friendship.

Personal Recollections

High Scientific Quality

Catherine Dacou-Voutetakis, Greece

A good many years have passed since my first attendance of an ESPE Annual Meeting. It was so very important for every young endocrinologist to attend these meetings and, especially, to make a presentation.

I very vividly recall my initial oral presentation in Bergen in 1973, following which Prof. Prader, looking most pleased, congratulated me. Standing quite nervous, I was delighted to hear him saying that I should become a member of the Society, and that he would support my candidacy. So, the following year I was elected an active member, something which we young scientists regarded as quite prestigious. Since then I have attended almost all the meetings and have observed what a great metamorphosis they have undergone over the years, not only in numbers but also in other aspects.

The Annual Meetings have always been of high scientific quality, which has followed an impressively ascending scale, primarily thanks to the efforts of the excellent General Secretaries to whom we must express our deep gratitude. Nevertheless, we must acknowledge that the meetings of the early years had that certain conviviality and warmth which, in recent years, because of the growing numbers of attendees, has somewhat faded. In the early days, on the day after the scientific meeting we would take off on an excursion, usually to really nice places, during which there was a lot of discussion that was not always on medical matters.

The gala dinners were outstanding, and most amusing anecdotes were told by different people. Let me recount just one of them that was related to the town of Bergen by Professor Ettore Rossi. 'I was walking around the town,' he said, 'and met a sweet little boy.' I asked him "Does it rain here all the time?" and the boy replied "I don't know, sir: I am only 8 years old".'

At every Annual Meeting we try to uncover the well-kept secret: the Prader award winner. What always gives the winner away is an impressive change of dress code: the tie, the suit. Last year I immediately spotted Ze'ev Hochberg.

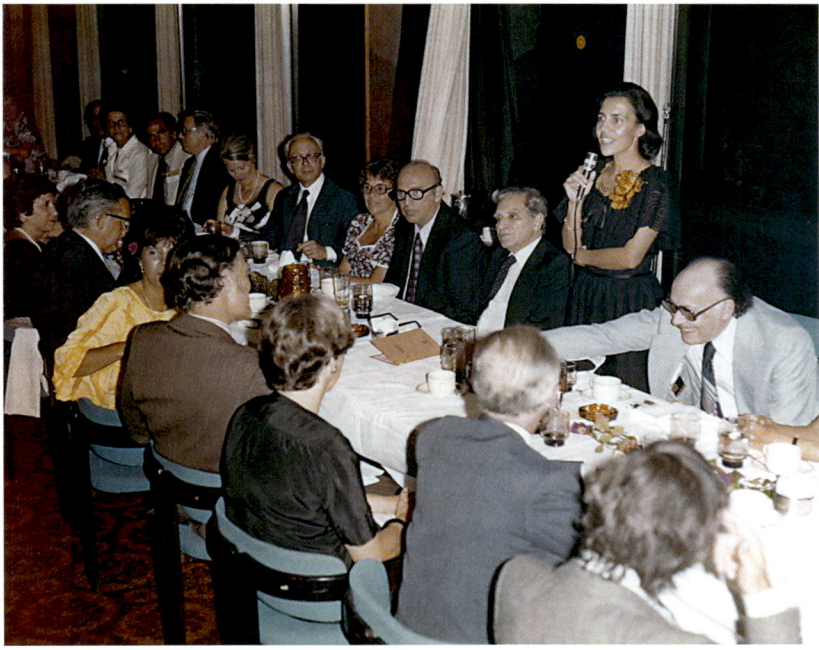

The gala dinner of the ESPE meeting in Vouliagmeni, which took place by a nice pool. Some of our beloved teachers and pioneers of ESPE are there: A. Prader, N. Matsaniotis, J. Tanner, H. Visser, M. New, A. M. DiGeorge and others. In my after dinner speech I included an explanation of the etymology of the word hermaphroditism. It has a charming myth explaining the mechanisms involved.

When Milo Zachmann was General Secretary I asked him about organising an ESPE meeting in Athens, one of the strongest point being the famous Greek weather. Milo was very much in favour and brought the proposal before the General assembly. Things were then much simpler and, fortunately, I did not have to make a presentation like the ones taking place now. The proposal was enthusiastically accepted by the General assembly. Thus, we undertook the quite heavy task of organizing the meeting in Athens in 1978 (so many years ago). In those days we did not have experienced congress organising companies like today, and the responsibility was mainly on the shoulders of the local organising committee.

The day before the scientific meeting in Athens, instead of a simple evening cocktail we went on a day cruise and stopped at two wonderful islands where we admired the beautiful blue sea. The day after the meeting we made an excursion to Epidaurus. Quite unexpectedly, the Bergen weather came along with us; it was pouring all day long. However, despite the heavy rain some dared to get off the bus and walk to the famous Epidaurus theatre with its exceptional acoustics and the Asklepieion, the sanctuary of Asklepius.

I must mention that while the organisation of the Athens meeting was in its final stage, Maria New called me to propose a roundtable discussion on congenital adrenal hyperplasia (CAH) so as to present the newly acquired data that the locus for the 21-hydroxylase gene was on the short arm of chromosome 6. Other highly interesting lectures concerned the DiGeorge syndrome presented by A.M. DiGeorge himself, the role of melatonin in humans, steroids in the brain, data on oral insulin, etc.

My involvement in other ESPE activities included participation in a committee on the use of growth hormone, in the Andrea Prader prize committee and in a committee for the training of paediatric endocrinologists in Europe. The latter formulated guidelines for the training program in paediatric endocrinology, and the criteria for the selection of trainees and the training centres. One of our primary objectives was the recognition of paediatric endocrinology as a subspecialty in the European Union.

In 2005, the Turner Syndrome (TS) Working Group was formed. I was one of the founding members and a coordinator until 2010. The symposia organized by this group enjoyed very good attendance and, most significantly, considerably improved our knowledge on the management of girls with TS. The same group initiated two projects, one on 'TS data recording in Europe' and another one on 'the use of very small doses of estrogens in the prepubertal period' as a possible preventive measure of osteoporosis and cardiovascular pathology.

I was also a founding member of the PAG (Paediatric and Adolescent Gynaecology) working group, proposed by Charles Sultan and a founding member of the GPED (Global Paediatric Endocrinology and Diabetes), established on the initiative of Ze'ev Hochberg, the mission being 'to improve the care of children in developing countries with endocrine disorders through the provision of training and educational opportunities, developing research and promoting advocacy for our goals.'

As might be expected, my fondest memory of ESPE is the meeting in 2007 in Finland in which I was given the Outstanding Clinician Award, which gave me the deepest scientific satisfaction ever.

Personal Recollections

Sippell WG (ed): ESPE – The First 50 Years. A History of the European Society for Paediatric Endocrinology.
Basel, Karger, 2011, pp 79–80

Integration and Globalisation

Feyza Darendeliler, Turkey

I have been working in the field of paediatric endocrinology for more than 15 years. I have been a member of ESPE since 1991. I have an interest in all fields of paediatric endocrinology, with special emphasis on growth, puberty, adrenal and growth disorders. I have always been interested in collaborative work and have participated in several multi-centre studies in Turkey and in Europe. Being an ESPE member has given me a chance to further collaborate with colleagues both on clinical grounds and personal academic grounds. ESPE means more to paediatric endocrinologists coming from outside the core 'European Union' countries. It means integration to the scientific know-how of developed countries, even before political integration can be achieved.

I remember the first ESPE meeting that I participated in in Copenhagen in 1988. It was a very exciting experience and a privilege to listen to and meet the leading paediatric endocrinologists of those years. There were very few of us from Turkey who participated in ESPE meetings at the time. Since then, with increasing globalisation and internet-access, and ESPE's approach and policy to become 'the' leading society in the field of paediatric endocrinology in the world, the number of colleagues from Turkey has increased to over 40 members.

Being elected as a member to the ESPE council from Turkey in 2009 is one of the highest achievements of my professional career. It is an honour for me, and I think it was made possible through the ESPE policy.

In the era of the political and cultural expansion of the European Union, I believe that it is critical to accompany such tremendous change with a scientific extension, which would allow the peripheral Europe to voice its concerns, benefit from the know-how of Old Europe and rise to the awaiting challenges with a more enlightened, healthy and integrated frame of mind. Since its foundation, ESPE has played a vital role in promoting research and training in the field of paediatric endocrinology in Europe. ESPE has reached its present esteemed position in the European and international paediatric community as a result of the hard and ambitious work of the ESPE administrators over the years. To maintain ESPE standards and to realize ESPE objectives, it is important that the present and future Council members have an equally ambitious and devoted outlook as their predecessors. In this context, those who laid the foundation stones of paediatric endocrinology in Europe must always be remembered and appreciated. I personally would like to include Olcay Neyzi in this list, since she has been the leading academic paediatric endocrinologist in Turkey for decades and continues to be the supportive force behind many of us who are working and publishing in the field of paediatric endocrinology. Prof. Neyzi has been my mentor throughout my academic career in Turkey, and she has especially provided support and guidance for me in reaching out from Turkey to the international arena of paediatric endocrinology.

Today, particularly in clinical research, multi-centred studies are gaining more and more importance. Cooperation in research leads to greater emphasis on evidence-based conclusions and also to cooperation in training activities, hence to an improvement in standards. Activities such as the ESPE Summer School, ESPE Winter School and all the scientific courses and meetings serve this purpose of integrating developing country practitioners into the scientific circle of established developed country professionals. This integration and globalisation brings a union of cultures, a deeper insight and a more fruitful collaboration. These activities have also led to the initiation or continuation of many friendships.

ESPE is indeed *the* paediatric endocrine society for those of us who are trying to find a balance in their work between basic research and clinical practice, between being a scientist and a clinical doctor, as well as between European Union countries and the rest of the world.

Personal Recollections

The ESPE Annual Meeting Concerts

Stenvert Drop, The Netherlands

Evening concerts during the annual meeting of ESPE have been a longstanding tradition. It has been a very wise initiative of the founding fathers of ESPE. I remember many of them, highly diverse, often with a local flavour, but always enjoyable.

One of the first suggestions, clearly non negotiable and indisputable, of my boss Professor Henk Visser was to attend ESPE Annual Meetings. Thus, my first ESPE meeting was in June 1979 in Ulm. I do not remember, I have to admit, the scientific sessions or the guided poster tours but I remember the concert. It was an organ recital, very static and serene, in the dark and freezing cold Münster of Ulm. At the end of the concert with music of Buxtehude, Bach and Franck and far away on the balcony in front of the organ there was the silhouette of the organist taking the hesitant applause of the ESPE audience.

In 1981, during the first Joint meeting in Geneva organized by Pierre Sizonenko, the String Quartet 'Quatuor de Genève' performed in the Piaget Hall of the University. As an amateur string player my recollection is biased by a non-suppressible feeling of 'Schadenfreude', as the first violinist got lost in the notoriously difficult fugue of the last movement of the Dissonant quartet by Mozart.

In 1982, I had my first oral presentation in Helsinki, but I remember mostly that two children of Professor Perheentupa performed on the violin and piano and the evening concert one day later was given by a charming youth orchestra and chorus. In Copenhagen in 1988 a chamber string ensemble played Mozart and the Holberg suite by Grieg with a beautiful and distinct viola part. In 1989 we attended in Jerusalem a performance entitled 'Wein, Weib und Gesang' of a band and a choir with Israeli music. In fact, during the months preceding the meeting there was a very lively postal exchange (emails did not exist) on having a performance of an orchestra consisting of just ESPE members and directed by its Secretary Ieuan Hughes. In spite of Zvi Laron's perseverance the idea did not crystallise for many logistical reasons.

At Palais Ferstel in Vienna 1992, the string soloists of the Vienna Philharmonic accompanied their first cellist in a tantalizing performance of the C major cello concerto by Haydn. In 1991, the meeting was in Berlin and the concert was in the Konzerthaus am Gendarmenmarkt. It was a very special concert not only as the hall was very beautiful, restored fully in accordance with the style and acoustics of the Musikvereinssaal in Vienna but also because of the choice of music. Joachim Pliquett (trumpet) and Arvid Gast (organ) gave a recital ranging from baroque to contemporary music. The sponsoring pharmaceutical company surprised all attendants with a CD, announced as the first of a long-lasting tradition but this CD is the only one in my possession.

In 1994, I was a member of the local organizing committee of the meeting in Maastricht. We had extensive discussions on the format of the concert and the choice of the program. We finally agreed to invite the Netherland Wind ensemble. On the program were songs by Moussorgsky with a Russian baritone. Just one week ahead we received a call that he could not come. However, increasing his honorarium appeared to solve the problem. It was a beautiful and moving concert with the Dvorak wind serenade as a very joyful finale.

In 1995 in Edinburgh with exceptionally beautiful sunny weather every day, the concert was given by the Hebrides string ensemble with music of Mozart and Dvorak. In 1996, it was again an organ recital in the 14th century St. Pierre Cathedral of Montpellier. During the Annual meeting in Warsaw in 1999, we heard a piano recital, of course with works of Chopin in a church where Chopin also used to perform. In 2000, the concert was given in the cathedral of Bruxelles with Bach cantatas. It had to be given twice because of the large number of ESPE meeting attendants. In 2003, the concert was part of the social event and was given in a cave outside of Ljubljana. The concert lasted only 30 minutes because the low temperature prevented the string players from playing any longer.

In 2006, the meeting was held in the 'Doelen' in Rotterdam, the home base of the Rotterdam Philharmonic Orchestra. It was a great pleasure to organise a concert in the main hall of the Doelen given by the Rotterdam chamber orchestra. They gave a thrilling performance of the 8th string quartet by Shostakowich and the Symphonia concertante for violin and viola by Mozart was played with vigour and tenderness by top soloists.

ESPE Annual meetings are nowadays attracting thousands of participants and logistics and resources limit the options for ESPE concerts. Still the initiative of the founding fathers is to be honoured. Following a long and hectic day of science it is not only relaxing but also comforting and unifying to enjoy live music performed by professional artists, just for you and your ESPE friends.

The Future of Paediatric Endocrinology in Spain Is Guaranteed

Angel Ferrández Longás, Spain

During my stay at the Zurich Kinderspital from 1965 to 1971, I gained progressively more and more interest in paediatric endocrinology. With teachers like Andrea Prader, Milo Zachmann, Ruth Illig, Gertrud Mürset and its increasing scientific importance, it is easy to understand that after 4 years of general paediatrics I decided, with the approval of Prof. Prader, to dedicate myself entirely to this young subspeciality. At the beginning of the 1960s a selected group of paediatricians from many European countries, coordinated and directed by Andrea Prader, created the ESPE.

The ESPE Meeting in June 1973 in Bergen, Norway, is special to me because I was admitted as a member following Dr. Francés Antonin, the first Spanish ESPE member and one of the founders of the Society. Besides the scientific aspects of the Meeting, looking from my room at people playing football at 11 p.m. in full day light impressed me forever.

For me another important date related to the ESPE was 1992, when Zaragoza was the site of the Annual meeting. The date was no coincidence; we celebrated that year the 500th Anniversary of the discovery of America by C. Colon under the orders, economic support and protection of Isabel de Castilla and Fernando de Aragón.

Under the warm enthusiasm of ESPE during the 1970s, more and more Spanish paediatricians became interested in paediatric endocrinology. Such an interest gave rise to the Spanish Society for Paediatric Endocrinology starting its official activities in 1978 in Zaragoza. Now this open Society is and has been an active group of the ESPE with many members involved in different working areas. The future of paediatric endocrinology in Spain is guaranteed, because many young people in different Spanish hospitals are very interested in this subspeciality and this interest is greatly influenced by ESPE. I'm sure that Andrea Prader and the group of the ESPE founders would feel very happy and satisfied with its contribution to the impressive development, now extended to the world, of paediatric endocrinology. To him, his group of founders and a huge group of successors along the years, our most sincere gratitude.

Personal Recollections

Sippell WG (ed): ESPE – The First 50 Years. A History of the European Society for Paediatric Endocrinology.
Basel, Karger, 2011, pp 85–87

ESPE Has Been Like a Family

Annette Grüters-Kieslich, Germany

I still remember my first Annual ESPE Meeting in Athens in 1978 with Prof. Dacou-Voutetakis as President. Being still a student at the Medical school of the Free University Berlin I had finished my doctoral thesis work and had started newborn screening for congenital hypothyroidism in all newborns in the former West-Berlin. Immediately before I had visited Professor Ruth Illig at the Kinderspital Zurich, who had started nationwide newborn screening for Switzerland together with Prof. König in Bern in 1975/1976. I presented a poster on nocturnal prolactin secretion in pre-pubertal and pubertal boys, a short study which was supervised by my mentor Dr. Sigrun Korth-Schütz, who had also supervised my doctoral thesis on dehydroepiandrosterone sulfate in pre-term and full-term newborns. I was not only impressed by the scientific work that was presented, but also by the close friendship many people at that meeting (only around 300 at that time) seemed to have. And I enjoyed the participation in the social programme: a visit to the Acropolis and the cruise in the Ägäis. I remember that Prof Maria New, the mentor of Dr. Sigrun Korth-Schütz, missed the cruise ship on one of the little islands and needed to be brought back to the ship with a little boat and many shopping bags.

As you may have noticed, four women introduced me to ESPE: Dr. Sigrun Korth-Schütz, Prof. Maria New, Prof. Ruth Illig and Prof. Dacou-Voutetakis. I recall this because I believe that this was a kind of 'imprinting effect'.

Only a year later, in 1979, still being a student I had my first oral presentation at the Annual Meeting in Ulm, Germany. This was a terrifying moment when my boss Prof. Hans Helge at the first day of the meeting told me that already next day I was supposed to give a short talk in the recent results session on my observation that newborns, after prenatal disinfection of the mother, present with TSH elevations in newborn screening. After a sleepless night I gave the talk and could hardly answer when Prof. Prader, whom I had admired since I met him in Zurich, asked me a question.

ESPE therefore presented itself to me as a friendly scientific society with a natural integration of women and young students and young academics.

After two more Annual Meetings, in Bergamo and Helsinki, the next important meeting was the first Joint meeting in Geneva 1982 where I met Prof. Delbert Fisher and asked him if I could spend a research fellowship in his institute. I realized that besides being a renowned and excellent scientist he is also a very friendly and open-minded person, and so I spent my research fellowship from 1983 to spring 1984 with him and therefore missed the Annual Meeting in Budapest.

In the next 23 years I only missed one Annual Meeting, in Jerusalem, to my deep regret, because my daughter was then only 10 months old.

I am very thankful that I had the opportunity to participate in all these meetings. The scientific exchange in the whole field of paediatric endocrinology was extremely important for my growing responsibility for so many patients. Sometimes poster presentations gave the clue to solve difficult diagnostic situations – like the picture of a patient with Peutz-Jeghers syndrome and precocious pseudopuberty on a poster at the Joint meeting in San Francisco in 1993 which came immediately to my mind when only a few months later such a patient was presented to us in the outpatient clinic.

However, it was not only the many things I learned, it was also the many enthusiastic researchers with whom longstanding professional as well as personal relationships and friendships developed which I deeply appreciate. It was always like a family reunion to meet again at the Annual Meetings.

The special spirit of the first ESPE Summer School in 1987 near Toulouse is probably another experience that was important for bonding to ESPE and paediatric endocrinology. And this seems to be true also for many of my co-students like Olle Söder, Juliane Leger, Wieland Kiess, Werner Blum – to name only a few.

Therefore, I felt very honoured when, in 1995, I was asked to be a teacher in the Summer School in Blairquhan Castle in Scotland. Here I met Ze'ev Hochberg for the first time and I was impressed by his knowledge, his skilled presentation of the Year in Paediatric Endocrinology and his analytical thinking which was very instrumental for the discussions with the students. Only 2 years later, I was invited to join the Summer School steering committee and in 2000 I took over the position as chairperson from Maguelone Forest, another female paediatric endocrinologist who had impressed me ever since I first met her at the first Summer School near Toulouse.

It is not exaggerated when I state that I would not have missed the 8 years with the ESPE Summer School as teacher, steering committee member and chairperson for anything. The farewell evenings, when Malcolm Donaldson played the guitar and the teachers were singing together with the students coming from so many different countries and schools, are close to my heart. These experiences are now of great value to me as Dean of the largest medical school in Germany, which I want to develop into an international school and research institution, because I think that in remembrance of history, Germany, and especially Berlin, should embrace diversity.

Would I Criticise Anything About ESPE?
Scientific competition sometimes creates unpleasant situations and encounters, and of course I have come across such episodes in the last 32 years. However the number of people with deep integrity and loyalty among the ESPE members far exceeded these rare situations – I was close to writing: mutations! – and I therefore strongly believe that it was this environment that stimulated my scientific curiosity and interest in paediatric endocrinology. Meeting so many excellent female basic and clinical scientists encouraged me to pursue a career in endocrinology.

I would like to finish my short collection of memories with the statement: ESPE has always been like a family and I look forward to many family reunions to come.

Lucky and Privileged to Be a Member

Ieuan Hughes, UK

I had the privilege of being ESPE Secretary from 1988 to 1992, followed by being the honorary President of the Society for the Joint Meeting with the LWPES in San Francisco in 1993, hosted by Mel Grumbach as the meeting President. But, firstly, I recall my baptism at an ESPE meeting which I attended after completing endocrine training with Jeremy Winter in Canada. ESPE was not on my radar during those years when *the* endocrine meetings to attend in North America were the Society for Pediatric Research (SPR) and, of course, The Endocrine Society. The 1977 ESPE meeting was held in Cambridge under the Presidency of Charles Brook. Not only was this my baptism in ESPE matters, but it was my first visit to Cambridge and my first encounter with Charles Brook. I'm not sure which one was most awe-inspiring! I recall the use of ancient lecture venues around the town (Cambridge celebrated its 800th birthday in 2009!), the beauty of the Colleges and the traditional ESPE concert held in King's College Chapel, no less. I still remember the concert given by the renowned English Chamber Orchestra included Mozart's Piano Concertos No. 27 and 11 played by Murray Perahia. Charles must have been very well connected! The scientific programme was also good and it was the first opportunity to present data on 17OH-progesterone profiles in congenital adrenal hyperplasia that we had collected during studies in Canada. I seemed to recall some vociferous discussion of our findings during the 5 minutes of questions, but survived that ordeal to become hooked on ESPE as a must Society to join. Little did I also realise at the time that I would be returning to Cambridge 12 years later to work in the University Department of Paediatrics.

Fast forward 10 years to when I 'shadowed' Al Aynsley-Green as Secretary for a year until taking over in 1988. Al had run a tight ship, superbly organised and it was with some trepidation that he was a difficult act to follow. Indeed, the first 'crisis' soon arose when the planned host centre for the 1988 meeting withdrew at short notice due to unforeseen circumstances. Even 23 years ago, organising the Annual Meeting of

ESPE was a major affair and very fortunately for the Society, Niels Skakkebaek volunteered to step into the breach to host the meeting in Copenhagen. What an outstanding show he put on. One need not have worried that Niels and his colleagues would ensure that, against all odds, the meeting would be a great success. Niels is very much a man of principle and I recall he did not take too kindly to an industry-sponsored pack of delegates arriving unannounced at the Panum Institute, expecting to be welcomed with open arms. Niels had other ideas! This episode spawned a lengthy debate on the links between the Society and the pharma industry, a relationship which today is mature and works in symbiosis to the good of paediatric endocrinology.

1989 was one of the most monumental years in the history of the ESPE, in my view. This was a joint meeting with LWPES which ESPE was hosting, not in Europe, but in Jerusalem with Zvi Laron as President. What a unique setting and how fortunate for both Societies and the many other delegates from around the world that we were able to meet then in safety in the Middle East which has seen, and continues to see, so much turmoil in its troubled history. Sadly, it was not possible to repeat the exercise of an Israel-based meeting in Haifa years later, the conference being transferred to Basel under the continued Presidency of Ze'ev Hochberg. By the time of the Jerusalem meeting, I was beginning to get in to my stride as Secretary. However, nothing had prepared me for working with Zvi! What a bundle of energy brimming with ideas. I soon learned to my cost that an off-the-cuff remark to Zvi would register, be morphed in to something big and announced with a fanfare. What do I mean? I happened to mention (probably relaxing too much over a glass of wine or two after a long Council meeting) that it would be fun one day to form an ESPE orchestra (since it was so traditional each year to have the ESPE concert). Within days almost of this Council meeting, each member of the Society received a letter (this was pre-email!) from Zvi as President announcing that the inaugural concert of the ESPE orchestra would be held during the Joint Meeting in Jerusalem under the baton of our Secretary, Ieuan Hughes! Members should contact Ieuan to indicate the instrument they played. Not daunted by the practicalities of humping cellos, double-basses, trombones and the like all the way to Jerusalem, Zvi would arrange local hire of such instruments! An urgent phone call was needed to temper Zvi's enthusiasm and to nip the idea in the bud before it seriously took hold! An ESPE choir would be a more practical option perhaps in future! Needless to say, the Jerusalem meeting was just fantastic, scientifically and culturally, and preceded by a Summer School held on a kibbutz on the shores of Lake Galilee. The 1989 Joint Meeting was some experience!

The second 3 years of my tenure as Secretary encompassed annual meetings in Vienna, Berlin and Zaragoza. The Berlin meeting under the Presidency of Volker Hesse in 1991 was held a mere two years after the fall of the Berlin Wall, a date vividly remembered for me personally (November 9th) as it coincided with my birthday. I had visited the former East in the early 1980s and could not then foresee any chance that the divisions in Germany and Berlin would ever be resolved. The 1991, ESPE meeting was a cause for celebration.

The Joint Meeting in 1993 was a wonderful occasion because that champion of Paediatric Endocrinology, Mel Grumbach, was in the driving seat. My role as representing ESPE was straightforward... just do as you are told! Of course in every Joint Meeting, a degree of friendly sparring takes place as each Society (and now there are several at the banqueting table) jostle for positions to ensure suitable representation for Plenary and Symposium speakers and topics, as well as the Chairs.

What else stands out in my memory worthy of highlighting in this great Society of ours? Educational and research opportunities have multiplied and flourished. The Summer and Winter Schools are successfully spawning serial generations of endocrinologists who cement life-long friendships, as indeed does the main meeting itself. Never will I forget the dawn excursion we had during a Summer School held on the island of Föhr, one of the German Friesian Islands in the North Sea and where Dr. Frederik Paulsen, founder of Ferring Pharmaceuticals had a family home. We had been instructed to dress appropriately for a walk across the mudflats to another island (Amrum) while the tide was low. That advice was not accurately heeded by one scholar from Bulgaria who turned up immaculately attired in a suit whose trousers soon became the worse for wear when the wading phase of the walk kicked in! He coped admirably through his delightful sense of humour.

It was a pleasure to be involved in establishing the Andrea Prader Prize, with the early recipients being recognised during Professor Prader's lifetime. My goodness, wouldn't he and his co-founding fathers of the Society be proud of what can be seen now 50 years later in terms of the magnitude of the Society itself, all the myriad activities and the role it plays as *the* premier paediatric endocrine society. Indeed as I write about personal recollections of my favourite scientific society, I am taking my turn as one of the tutors based in the Nairobi African Paediatric Endocrine Centre. Now who would have thought that from its inception, ESPE 50 years later, together with other relevant Societies, would be spreading its wings to enable paediatric endocrine and diabetes services to begin to flourish in this great continent. I have indeed been very lucky and privileged to be a member of such a wonderful and rewarding Society.

The Impact of ESPE on Paediatric Endocrinology in Slovenia and Its Surroundings

Ciril Krzisnik, Slovenia

Paediatric endocrinology was introduced in Slovenia in 1960 by Prof. Dr. Leo Matajc who, after the visit to Prof. Henry Lestradet in Paris, started to treat diabetic children adapting the doses of insulin to results of self management based on measurement of glycosuria and ketonuria, and later glycaemia. In Ljubljana, three growth hormone-deficient patients started to be treated by growth hormone extracted from human pituitary glands – the procedure had already been done in the USA in 1968.

Attending the meetings of the International Study Group on Diabetes in Children and Adolescents (ISGD), I had the opportunity to meet some paediatric endocrinologists who were also members of ESPE. Thus I got information about ESPE and I attended the ESPE/LWPS meeting in 1981 in Geneva (with an invitation from Alan Drash and Salvatore Raiti) in connection with the ISGD meeting in Les Collones in the Swiss Alps close to Geneva.

Since then I have always had the possibility to attend the ESPE meetings where I could meet many colleagues and join different activities. After a visit of Ruth Illig from Zurich we introduced neonatal screening of congenital hypothyroidism in Ljubljana in 1981, the whole of Slovenia was covered in 1984. We followed the patients using the modified Zurich protocol and used the ESPE guidelines to monitor and treat these patients.

Together with Zvi Laron, we investigated hereditary dwarfism families on the island Krk and cooperated with him in investigations in diabetes and growth hormone resistance.

Later on we started intensive research collaboration within the so called 'Middle-European' ESPE countries together with Zelmira Misikova/Bratislava, Herwig Frisch/Vienna, Ferenc Péter/Budapest, Jan Lebl/Prague.

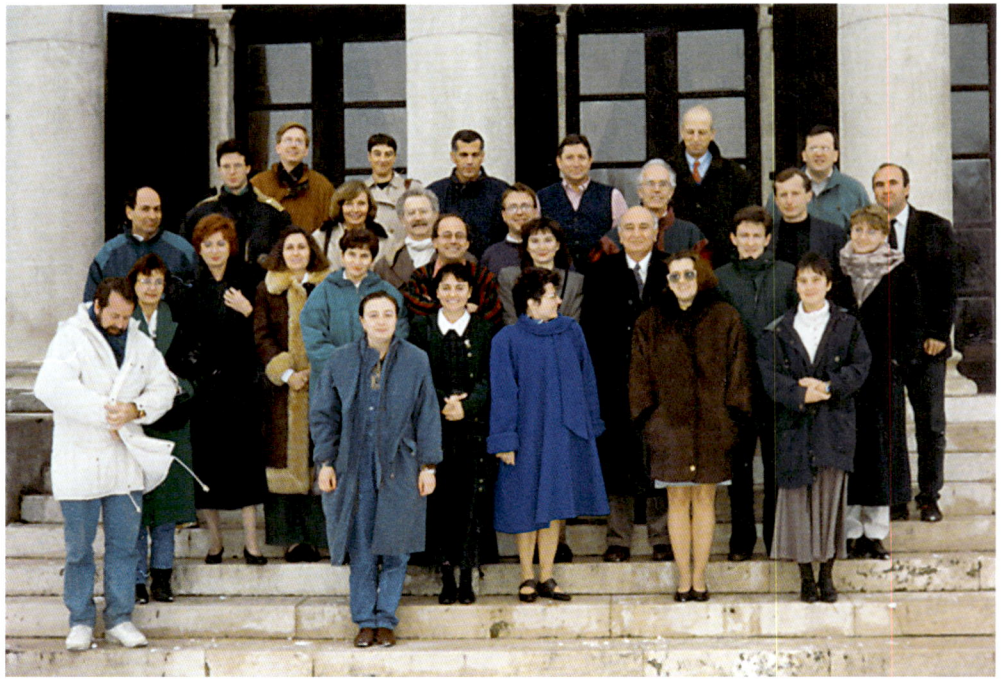

First ESPE Winter School in Hungary – December 1995.

As the number of paediatric endocrinologists in Slovakia, Austria, Hungary, Czech Republic and Slovenia was small and did not exceed 60, we decided to form the MESPE – Middle European Society of Paediatric Endocrinology which somehow replaced national paediatric endocrinological societies.

The joint studies of this group on CAH and thyroid disorders were presented at ESPE meetings. Some of the studies had recruited patients from the more than 60 millions of inhabitants in these five countries which increased the value of our investigations. The impact of Prof. Herwig Frisch, 'the spiritus movens' in this collaboration within Central and Eastern Europe, has been immense.

Together with Zvi Laron, Christos Bartsocas, Charles Sultan and Olcay Neyzi we also arranged a collaboration with paediatric endocrinologists in the Mediterranean area: Egypt, Israel, Turkey, Greece, Bulgaria, Serbia, Montenegro, Macedonia, Bosnia, Croatia, Slovenia, Italy, France and Spain.

The ESPE Winter and Summer Schools were very important for the education of young doctors focussing on paediatric endocrinology. I want to mention that we participated in the ESPE Winter School in Hungary in Seregélyes in 1995 which was organized by Ze'ev Hochberg, Paul Czernichow, Martin Ritzén, Wolfgang Sippell, Jean-Pierre Bourguignon, Pierre Chatelain and Ferenc Péter.

Many young doctors who participated in this meeting have meanwhile become leaders in the field of paediatric endocrinology in their region. Six years later, we organized the ESPE Summer School in Bled preceding the 42nd Annual Meeting of ESPE which we organized in Ljubljana in 2003.

The collaboration with ESPE members played an important role in clinical work and research in the field of paediatric endocrinology in Slovenia. Paul Czernichow in Paris hosted Tadej Battelino as research fellow in his department and laboratory. Prof. Battelino later introduced diagnostic procedures in molecular biology and genetics at the University Children's Hospital in Ljubljana which significantly improved clinical and research work in our area. Dr. Mojca Tansek got her clinical experience at the University Children's Hospital in Bergen, Norway (Prof. Aarskog), Primoz Kotnik has been engaged in research of nephrogenic diabetes insipidus at the institute run by Prof. Jakob Nielsen in Aarhus in Denmark, and Dr. Magdalena Avbelj has done research on idiopathic hypogonadotropic hypogonadism at Harvard University in Boston with W. F. Crowley.

Another important cooperation took place with Martin Savage enabling us to participate in the research programme on growth hormone insensitivity syndrome. Martin Ritzén has encouraged us to form the Prader Willi syndrome association in Slovenia (IPWSO) in order to do research on this genetic disorder and to help these patients and their families. Research and collaboration in paediatric diabetology has continued with Moshe Phillip/Israel, especially in the development of insulin pump treatment and closed loop insulin devices.

In conclusion, we can state that ESPE has directly and indirectly very much improved the treatment, care and research in children and adolescents suffering from endocrine disorders in Slovenia and the surrounding countries.

What ESPE Means to Me

Zvi Laron, Israel

In 1962 on a Swissair plane to the Netherlands to an endocrine meeting in Nordvijk I happened to sit near Andrea Prader, whom I met for the first time. He told me that after that meeting and following the Acta Endocrinologica Congress in Geneva (July 1962) he had invited all European paediatric endocrinologists attending that congress to Zurich for an informal scientific exchange of ideas. He invited me too, learning that I had established the first paediatric endocrine clinic in Israel. I accepted wholeheartedly and so came to know the early birds in paediatric endocrinology in Europe and start a lifetime of connections, collaboration and friendship.

The encounter in Zurich, which took place at the Kinderspital, discussed mainly growth problems and the use of anabolic steroids as growth stimulants. It was also a short time after the first publication by Maurice Raben on the use of pituitary extracted human growth hormone. This meeting in July 1962 was the foundation of what was to subsequently become the European Society for Paediatric Endocrinology (ESPE).

We were housed at the Eos hotel (nicknamed Eros for the parties given by Ruth Illig). I shared the room with Henk Visser and I remember that in his company I spent two sleepless nights; the first was in Zurich when we discussed our families and Mid-Eastern politics and became close friends until the present. The second night was at the Visser's home in Rotterdam, watching Armstrong step on the moon in 1968 (Margaret, his wife, finally went to bed leaving us with plenty of wine and Dutch cheese). Henk Visser organized the 2nd meeting in Groningen in 1963 and since then ESPE meets yearly and has grown from a Club to a European Society and then to a real International Society with many scientific and educational activities.

It was the model and stimulus to the founding of other national and regional paediatric endocrinology societies, including the Lawson Wilkins Pediatric Endocrinology Society (now named PES – Pediatric Endocrinology Society) in 1972 [1].

I have attended all ESPE Meetings since 1962 and had the honor to be its President twice. In 1967 I organized the meeting in Haifa (Israel) and the 2nd time in 1989 as President of the 4th joint ESPE-LWPES Meeting in Jerusalem. The last was attended by 900 participants, among them for the first time representatives of regional Paediatric Endocrine Societies.

In addition to providing a platform to present scientific novelties, the ESPE Meeting provided the opportunity to meet not only colleagues but to get to know their family members, to visit their homes and, with many, to start friendly connections.

The only disappointment I found in the first years was the disinterest in diabetes mellitus, a disease with an increasing incidence in modern society. I had many discussions on this topic with Andrea Prader, but not until Eugen Schoenle became Head of Endocrinology was this truly implemented in Zurich. This issue led me to initiate with Henry Lestradet in Paris (interested in diabetes but not in general endocrinology) and Helmuth (Jean) Loeb in Bruxelles, the founding of a separate society in 1974, first named ISGD (International Study Group for Diabetes in Children) and which changed its name to ISPAD (International Pediatric and Adolescent Diabetes Society) in 1993.

To my great satisfaction in recent years ESPE members and organizers have incorporated diabetes mellitus in the Annual Meeting Program and the relationship between the two societies has led to joint programs.

Getting older, but still active, I do not know how many more meetings I shall be able to attend; certainly not the 75th Anniversary.

ESPE, its founders, members, families and meetings have meant and still mean much to me. Personal friendships, meeting colleagues beyond political boundaries, inspiration for research, connection with the pharma industry, etc. A long and happy relationship.

Congratulations ESPE and its young leadership and wishing ESPE Many Happy Returns on the occasion of its 50th birthday.

Reference

1 Fisher DA, Laron Z: The early history of paediatric endocrinology. Pediatr Endocrinol Rev 2003;1 (suppl 1):66–91.

A Long Way to ESPE from Behind the 'Iron Curtain'

Jan Lebl, Czech Republic

One of the basic principles of the communist regimes in Central Europe was keeping people inside and not allowing them to travel out to the non-communist world, to prevent them from meeting people from other countries and bringing back new stimuli 'contaminated by the fresh air of freedom'. The situation might have been slightly better in Poland and Hungary; from the former Czechoslovakia, however, just the most loyal members of the Communist Party occasionally received permission to participate in international medical meetings in Western Europe or overseas. As there were no loyal communists among paediatric endocrinologists, contacts with ESPE did not exist at all.

The first Czech to become an ESPE member was Olga Hnikova who, in the late 1980s, was invited to join the society by Prof. Ruth Illig. Prof. Illig supported her in developing neonatal screening for congenital hypothyroidism which came into effect in Czechoslovakia in 1985.

Just a little substitute for participation at ESPE meetings were occasional workshops in East Germany and in Hungary with participation of colleagues coming from Western European countries. Especially the East German meetings were attended by several prominent paediatric endocrinologists. For me and my friend and co-worker Stanislava Kolousková, the most inspiring experience was attending a workshop in Magdeburg in 1988 and discussing growth hormone therapy with Michael Ranke, iodine deficiency with Francois Delange and prenatal treatment of congenital adrenal hyperplasia with Maguelone Forest.

The fall of the iron curtain in 1989 was some kind of a miracle. The world re-opened and friendly people who were coming from 'behind' were waiting to meet us. In fact, the pharmaceutical companies were the first to help overcome the financial barriers and facilitate participation in international meetings. I will remember the first one forever - a Kabi meeting on growth hormone held in Edinburgh in April 1990, with the programme carefully compiled by Rolf Gunnarsson. At that one, as well as at many additional meetings, I was impressed by the friendly and collaborative atmosphere of the international community of paediatric endocrinologists that I still deeply esteem.

The essential step forward to ESPE was initiated by our collaboration with colleagues from Austria, facilitated by Herwig Frisch. Thanks to the support of the Schwarzenberg Foundation in Vienna, I worked together with Herwig's team in 1992. I learned how to efficiently conduct clinical research and how to write scientific articles and transmitted these new skills to my co-workers in Prague. In subsequent years, a couple of them came to work temporarily in Vienna thanks to Austrian governmental support. In 1993, we together with Herwig Frisch and Ciril Krzisnik, opened a series of 'Middle-European Workshops on Paediatric Endocrinology', challenging all of us to make ready talks and presentations in English and to actively discuss clinical and scientific issues of our patients. The 'MEWPE' countries finally included Austria, Slovenia, Czechia, Slovakia and Hungary.

Ze'ev Hochberg visited Prague in 1995, being the first official ESPE emissary when looking for locations for the first ESPE Winter School. Finally he decided on Seregélyes, Hungary. However, Winter School came to Prague just a bit later, in 2000, under the supervision and careful organization of Henriette Delemarre-van der Waal and with participation of Leo Van den Brande, Charles Sultan, Anatolij Tjulpakov and some other teachers. Winter Schools bring stimulation to both students and teachers. We all remember Leo Van den Brande teaching the principles of clinical research and of preparing presentations. He was proposing to arrange patient case reports as stories of a child's life, using its given name and including some details on his interests and hobbies, to introduce the human dimension of a medical report. Since then, we are holding biannual meetings of the Czech paediatric endocrine group over presentations of such case reports by all participants – as our little local heritage of Leo Van den Brande.

Chris Kelnar asked me in 2000 to consider joining the ESPE Clinical Fellowship committee. Two years later, he took over the chair of the committee and nominated me as the committee secretary at the ESPE annual meeting in Madrid. For me, Chris Kelnar became a great teacher of the British tradition of credibility and dignity. As the resources for clinical fellowships did not match with the needs of all the applicants that year, he considered and evaluated all applicants from all aspects, aiming to identify those who would most profit from the fellowship and would bring the knowledge and skills to his home institution to benefit the patients. Later, the two former fellows, Rasa Verkauskiene from Kaunas, Lithuania, and Violeta Iotova from Varna, Bulgaria, joined the committee and helped much in developing its mission. In nine years working for the committee, we took part in the gradual switch of ESPE from a society of Europe and the Mediterranean to an organization with global impact. We welcomed the first fellow from Latin America (Rafael Mantovani from Belo Horizonte, Brazil)

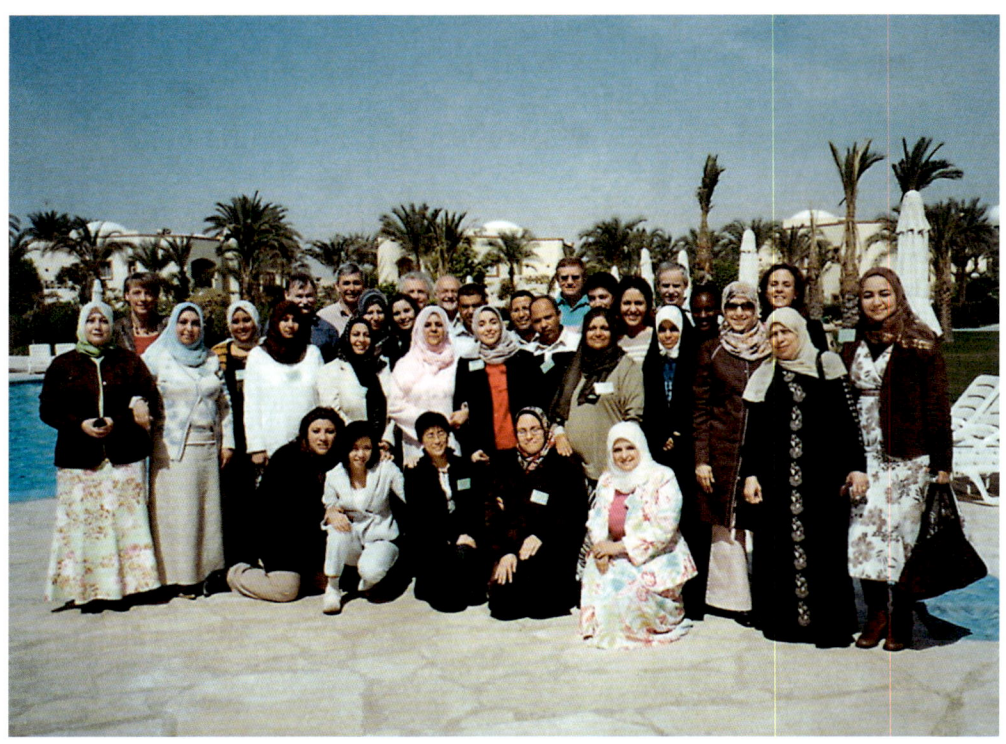

Students and teachers at ESPE Winter School in Ain Sukhna, Egypt, March 2008.

and from India (Sudha Rao Chandrashekhar from Mumbai) in a European training centre in 2005, followed by fellows from Pakistan, Tanzania, Kenya, Cameroon, Morocco, Tunisia, United Arab Emirates, China and some other countries in the subsequent years.

Winter Schools continue to be a great experience, and frequently initiate and stimulate life-long friendships. Of Winter Schools that I attended as a teacher or organiser (Moscow 1999, Prague 2000, Vilnius 2004, Dobógokö in Hungary 2005, Prague 2007, Ain Soukhna in Egypt 2008), the last one was undoubtedly the most impressive. Organised by the enthusiastic young paediatric endocrinologist Rasha Hamza from Cairo and chaired by Angela Hübner, it was attended by students arriving from half the globe starting in Morocco and ending in Thailand and China. The global community of students and teachers facilitated understanding the needs of young patients with diabetes and other endocrine conditions worldwide, regardless of the continent, religion or gross national product. And the friendly atmosphere was greatly underlined by Malcolm Donaldson's guitar in the late evenings, after all students' case presentations had been completed and discussed. Of all the songs from the countries of residence of the students, 'Malayka' from Tanzania, introduced by Edna Majaliwa, became the most popular.

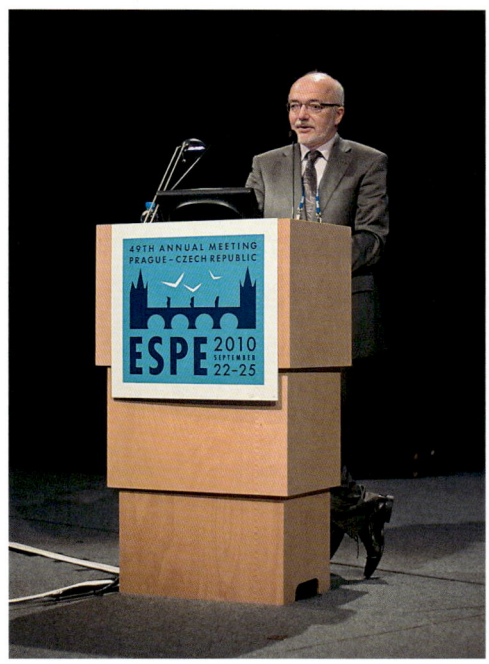 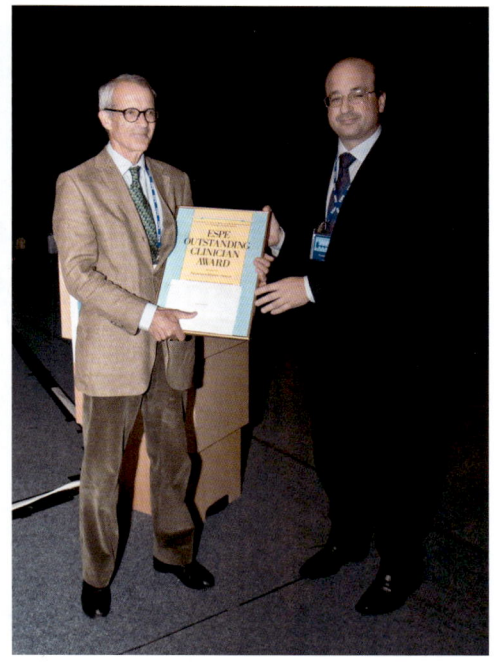

The opening talk of Jan Lebl at the 49th Annual ESPE meeting in Prague.

Herwig Frisch is accepting the Outstanding Clinician Award from Franco Chiarelli, ESPE Secretary General.

In 2010, the 20th year of liberty of Central-East and Eastern Europe, Prague became the capital of paediatric endocrinology, hosting the 49th Annual ESPE meeting. With 3,287 participants from 92 countries, it represented the largest ever paediatric endocrine meeting in Europe by the number of attendance. And even more – two of those who substantially contributed to overcoming the gap between former West and East Europe in paediatric endocrinology, were acknowledged by the major ESPE awards. The Andrea Prader Prize was awarded to Ze'ev Hochberg from Haifa, Israel. He is not only a brilliant researcher but also the inventor and founder of multiple ESPE educational programmes, including the ESPE Winter School, the Nairobi training centre project and others. Herwig Frisch from Vienna, Austria, received the Outstanding Clinician Award. Recognised as an excellent clinician, researcher and teacher, he has personally greatly contributed to re-unifying Europe within the past 20 years.

ESPE Turns 50: Many Happy Returns and Best Wishes from Switzerland

Primus Mullis, Switzerland

I feel deeply honoured to represent Switzerland and to congratulate our Society on its 50th anniversary on behalf of the Swiss Society for Paediatric Endocrinology and Diabetology.

Without doubt, ESPE is and remains 'my' society, of which I became a member in the 1980s. I always felt encouraged and stimulated within the Society. Through my activities (ESPE Clinical Fellowship Programme, Programme Organizing Committee, Advanced Seminar in Developmental Endocrinology, ESPE Research Unit and Summer School) I made many friends with whom I spent time, not only successfully talking about science, setting up experiments and collaborating, but also enjoying sporting activities in the mountains or on golf courses and leisure time.

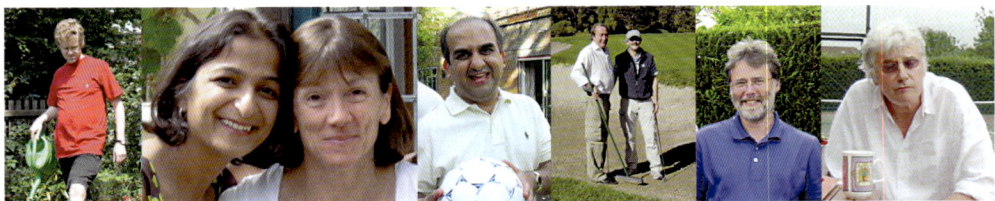

I remember well the 1986 meeting in Zurich, the 25th Annual Meeting, when Klaus Zuppinger, my mentor from Bern introduced me to Zvi Laron. I was astonished by his youthful appearance and, honestly, when I meet Zvi today, he still looks the same: I would like to know your recipe, Zvi!

In the late 1980s I moved to London where I joined Charles Brook's Department at the Middlesex Hospital in London, another important figure in ESPE. It was he who introduced me not only to 'my' field of research (Charles, I am so grateful for that) but also to all the ESPE activities. Although strong-minded and determined about his ideas and concepts, he has given me the freedom to develop my own ideas and concepts in the lab.

As always in life, there were people who had a striking impact on one's personal life, even without knowing it. Such exciting persons were Leo van den Brande and Jaako Perheentupa for me. They were always interested in the newest results and were, therefore, so stimulating to me as a young scientist and clinician.

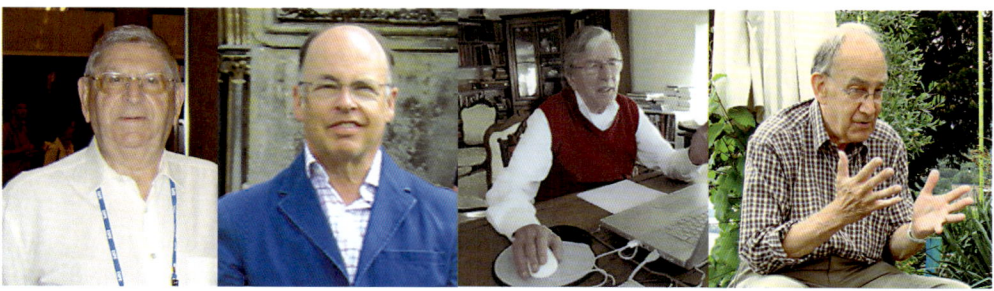

Three names from Switzerland stand out in ESPE history: Andrea Prader, Milo Zachmann and Pierre Sizonenko. These grand-seigneurs of Swiss Paediatric Endocrinology had a most powerful impact on what was going on in Switzerland and were supportive to all of us, but their contributions to ESPE were crucial.

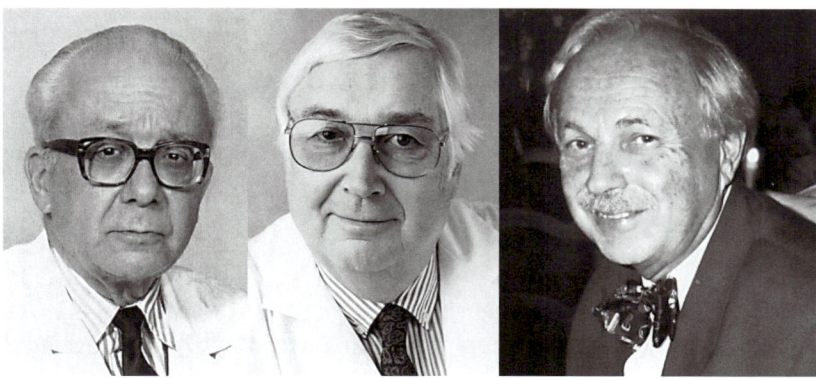

Andrea Prader, one of the most influential figures in European paediatrics, is a founding father of paediatric endocrinology and started ESPE. He described hereditary fructose intolerance, hypocalcaemic pseudo-vitamin D deficiency as a genetic type of rickets, Prader-Willi syndrome. His interest turned to adrenal cortical disorders and his work eventually led to a description of lipoid adrenal hyperplasia and the discovery of 17,20-lyase deficiency. He also made seminal contributions in the area of growth and puberty, growth hormone and paediatrics as a whole. The Zurich longitudinal growth study was a model of such undertakings.

He was well-known for his international lectures and was elected a member of the British Royal College of Paediatrics and other societies. He received honorary doctorates and prizes from several universities and The European Society for Paediatric Endocrinology created an annual award, the Andrea Prader Prize, which is given to a member who demonstrates leadership and accomplishment in the field of paediatric endocrinology.

Milo Zachmann, well known for his impact on steroids, adrenal gland and congenital adrenal hyperplasia. For many years his laboratory was the gold standard for steroid analysis in urine. The Zachmann 'profile' was stated and every paediatric endocrinologist knew what it stood for. Milo, who had been the Secretary of ESPE from 1972 to 1977, was the first recipient of the 'Andrea Prader Prize'. This Prize was given to Milo to recognise his outstanding leadership and overall contribution to the field of paediatric endocrinology.

Pierre Sizonenko was the generalist among the paediatric endocrinologists of his time. Based in Geneva, he created a most distinguished clinical as well as research setting and published in many fields, belonging to the opinion leaders within the field of paediatric endocrinology. He was the mentor and organiser of the first Joint Meeting with the Lawson Wilkins Pediatric Endocrine Society (LWPES) of North America.

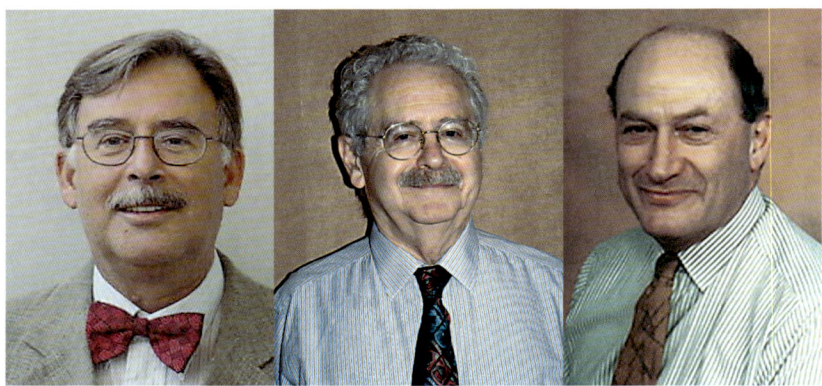

Finally, for me personally, I was much supported by many distinguished colleagues, who became friends over the years. Three I would like to highlight are Michael Ranke, during whose tenure as Editor-in-Chief of Hormone Research in Paediatrics, I became an associate editor. With Paul Czernichow, Olle Söder and Michel Polak, we started the 'ESPE Advanced Seminar in Developmental Endocrinology', which takes place each year, the purpose of which is to combine basic science and clinical paediatric endocrinology. Stephen Shalet, an adult endocrinologist but a longstanding member of the ESPE, was not only interested in my endocrine results, but also in the mountains I climbed.

In 2007, I received the ESPE Research Award in recognition of research achievements of outstanding quality in the fields of basic endocrine science or clinical paediatric endocrinology. I was and am still proud to be an ESPE member, thanks to all of you.

Personal Recollections

A Greek Adventure

Maria New, USA

ESPE was on a ship tour around Greece, stopping at various islands. I cannot remember the name of the particular island, but there was one where Lenore Levine and I decided to get off to do some shopping. We bought several lovely Greek skirts and became so engrossed in the shopping that we missed the little boat back to the ship. I then hired a fisherman's boat to rejoin the cruise and Lenore and I rowed back to the ship waiting for us so we could continue on the tour. Many people were laughing and taking pictures of these two women, Lenore and me, coming back on a fisherman's boat to join the cruise. Eyewitnesses reported that the boat was listing heavily to one side because everyone wanted to get a look!

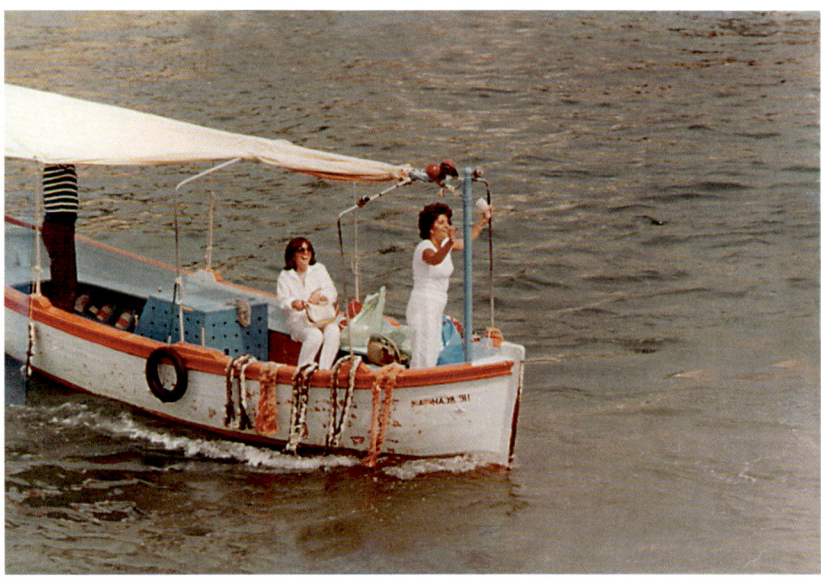

It was at that meeting that I met Dr. Miro Dumic, who later became a member of ESPE. He was very critical of these two wild American women who missed the ship and had to hire a fishing boat. Later, however, Dr. Dumic and I became close friends and collaborators. Indeed, Dr. Dumic discovered the famous case of an XY female who gave birth to a daughter. This was published in the JCEM and the ovaries made the cover of the JCEM because though the ovary was 46 XY and SRY positive, it had follicles [1]. So the trip had a happy ending!

Reference

1 Dumic M, Lin-Su K, Leibel N, Ciglar S, Vinci G, Lasan R, Nimkarn S, Wilson JD, McElreavey K, New MI: Report of fertility in a woman with a predominantly 46,XY karyotype in a family with multiple disorders of sexual development. J Clin Endo Metab 2008;93:182–189.

Personal Recollections

The Transition of ESPE

Raphaël Rappaport, France

The ESPE has reached half a century in age and has grown into an adult, serious well-recognized Society with thousands of participants from all over the world (even some Americans!) attending each meeting. Did we ever anticipate such a success story when the Founders met for the first time in Zurich in 1962? My mentor Professor Pierre Royer was among them and asked me to take over the lead and I joined the group the year after. This was a starting point to my career and to the development of paediatric endocrinology at my University. A few years later politics came into play in a quite surprising manner: Europe was still a dream and the French government who gave a grant for my participation at the ESPE meeting had decided that we could not accept English as the only official language. I was summoned to present my paper in French. I did so, nobody understood and the discussion was quite short. At least everybody knew that I was bilingual. Years later in 1977, in spite of this episode, the Council elected me to act as Secretary of the Society. After the Rotterdam meeting I took over from Milo Zachmann, a experienced and active frequent flyer (with his own plane) through all Europe. I certainly could not compete with the same weapons.

Actually it soon became clear to me that the ESPE was a young adolescent in the transition phase (according to present standards). We were still in the big well before reaching mature adulthood.

Believe it or not, one important issue at that time was the financing of the Society. France was nor secure enough to host our 'treasure'. The only partner we could trust was a Swiss bank. It happened that Pierre Sizonenko, a well-established colleague, accepted to act as treasurer in Geneva. With Pierre I had the most rewarding partnership, as in a family business. And it is true that at that time the Society still was a large family. We had to promote Pediatric Endocrinology in Europe, with new countries participating every year. The ESPE meeting was a distinct honour for the inviting venue and the President of the year was the 'local' and 'European' scientific organiser . . . with some help from the Council. Far from the Programme Organizing

Committee as you see it nowadays, the scientific content was out of the Council's control. In retrospect I think we did it well, leaving each inviting country the choice of topics and speakers with a large 'local' contribution. I suppose it helped promoting our speciality. And certainly it did not hurt our development. Here we were in a true 'transition' to a modern fully European society as it is today.

It took me several years to convince the ESPE council that we needed a programming scientific committee. As a result I was elected to chair the first of these POCs which are now central to the scientific policy of the Society. This was quite an experience in a cheerful and constructive atmosphere.

Convention centres like the ones we attend today were just being constructed all over Europe. Therefore, we had the unique opportunity to meet in venues like King's College next to the river Cam, the Apollon Palace Hotel near Athens (Apollon was a nice name!), Seminario Giovanni XXIII in the old Bergamo, and last but not least the Universities of Ulm, Geneva and Helsinki. Thanks to the presidents for their choices!

Each year the crowd was growing and we could foresee the coming change into a true European structure with more than a thousand attendants locked in air-conditioned convention centres. The great event of my term was the 1st ESPE-LWPES Joint Meeting, superbly organised by Pierre Sizonenko and Michel Aubert. The venue was the UNI in Geneva, and the scientific programme was the best we could afford at that time. Let us say that it probably was the last science-based event in our society with vast physiology approaches and new developmental topics before the coming explosion of molecular biology and genetics. Do not forget that our Swiss friends brought to the meeting a symbolic cow whose famous bell was given to the Society as a mark to be transmitted to all future Joint meetings. Do not forget that Swiss cows are vigorous uphill climbers . . . like all paediatric endocrinologists!

So the years went by for a fine, stimulating and responsible Society. I have had the unique opportunity to share this enterprise with all my friends for so many years, starting long ago . . .

Personal Recollections

Sippell WG (ed): ESPE – The First 50 Years. A History of the European Society for Paediatric Endocrinology.
Basel, Karger, 2011, pp 107–110

My ESPE: Personal Views and Memories of My Favourite Society

Martin Ritzén, Sweden

ESPE is reaching its 50 years anniversary. My favourite society and I have matured together. Most of the founders are not with us anymore, and members like me, who joined ESPE 10 years after the foundation, are retiring. But once a member of ESPE, you are apt to always stay a member! For the last 50 years, I have joined and enjoyed every single meeting of ESPE, while I have joined and left many others. ESPE has a special place in my heart.

In the beginning, my relation with ESPE was not easy. In short, it was difficult to be accepted! After a successful postdoc period with one of the foremost members of the American Paediatric Endocrinology 'Nobility' (the definition of this imaginary Nobility was that he/she had been a former fellow of Lawson Wilkins), Jud Van Wyk at Chapel Hill, North Carolina, I was convinced that I would be greeted with open arms by ESPE. However, at that time only members, accompanied by one guest, were allowed to take part in the meeting. Sweden had a single member (one of the 30 founders, Carl-Gustaf Bergstrand), and he already had another guest who was closer to him! Anyway, another senior Scandinavian member stepped in, and since 1971 I have almost been married to ESPE!

Young as I was and full of self-confidence, I presented the molecular cause of androgen insensitivity; absence of a functioning androgen receptor in an androgen-insensitive rat. The only comment from the audience to this breakthrough in science was the conclusion of the chairman – a Scottish profile in paediatric endocrinology and a founding member: 'This is very interesting, *if true*'! I was astounded! Of course it was true! At that time, ESPE meetings were mostly concerned with clinical matters and case reports. Most of the audience were not ready to comprehend basic science. Later, when I had become a member of the Council, I took part in the ever returning debates on whether ESPE should go more or less in a direction towards basic or clinical science. At that time there were no parallel sessions and all the 100–200 participants listened to everything. My later experience, not least during my 6 years as chairman of the Programme Organizing Committee, is that ESPE meetings have now reached a good balance between basic and clinical science lectures.

Over the last decades, a major part of new discoveries within biomedicine has come from America. This American dominance is, for example, demonstrated by the Nobel Prizes in Physiology or Medicine; more than half have gone to the USA, many of them to immigrants from Europe. While endocrinology at large is no exception, *paediatric* endocrinology has not followed the same path. This is displayed by the development of ESPE meetings that are now unquestionably the foremost annual forum for paediatric endocrinologists from all over the world. The later appearance of our American counterpart, the Lawson Wilkins Pediatric Endocrine Society (now called Pediatric Endocrine Society) has not challenged this position. The successful history of the ESPE meetings to become more and more international has not passed unopposed. Over many years, the Annual Business Meetings have witnessed long discussions on whether ESPE should remain a club for the invited and privileged, or be open to anyone active in paediatric endocrinology. The latter has now become the rule. ESPE membership is open for anyone who has proven activity in the field, irrespective of citizenship, within or outside Europe. ESPE is now the global centre of paediatric endocrinology.

ESPE members have always had very intimate relations with American colleagues. Many of the leading European paediatric endocrinologists have had a period of training in the USA. It was therefore logical to have a 'Joint meeting of ESPE and LWPES', occurring every 4 years on alternate sides of the Atlantic Ocean. This tradition was started by Pierre Sizonenko in 1981 in Geneva and has continued ever since. Paediatric endocrinologists from other parts of the world eventually became more and more frustrated at being left out, and some threatened to form 'The International Society for Paediatric Endocrinology', to compete with the Joint Meetings. When I got the honour to become the president of the 5th Joint Meeting of ESPE and LWPES in Stockholm in 1997, I proposed to call it 'International Congress of Paediatric Endocrinology', but I was over-ruled by my colleagues in the ESPE Council. As a compromise, the sister societies of South America, Australasia and Japan were invited to collaborate in the planning of the Joint Meetings. That organization is still prevailing.

In 1981, during a sabbatical leave in Sweden, Paul Czernichow and I met at the National Gallery in Stockholm. Paul had the idea that ESPE should pay more attention to the coming generation of European paediatric endocrinologists by organizing a 'Summer School' for a few days preceding each annual meeting. I thought it was a great idea, and the planning was initiated. The Summer School was started under Paul's leadership and has developed in a very successful way.

However, before the opening of the iron curtain in 1989, the central and eastern European countries had lagged behind in paediatric endocrinology, as in many other medical fields. Ze'ev Hochberg observed this, and proposed that ESPE should arrange a 1-week annual 'Winter School' in these countries. I had the privilege to teach at the first one in a cold and snowy Hungarian mansion. The busy schedule exhausted the fellows of the course, who actually went on strike, when after the second full day of lectures (in English, not well understood by all), a night session was to be set up on 'How to set up a clinical study'. This session was substituted by beer drinking and joking in the bar...

Great progress has now been made in the former communist countries. Thus, Ze'ev Hochberg again looked around and found that the knowledge of paediatric endocrinology in the Sub-Saharan African countries was almost non-existent. ESPE should help to spread the message! As a first attempt, ESPE Council asked me to lead a Winter School type course in Nigeria, in 2005. Five ESPE members made up the faculty. We met wonderful young paediatricians with good textbook knowledge of endocrinology but little clinical guidance. The course was applauded, but after we left nothing happened. It was evidently not the way to go in the future. Instead, Ze'ev (again) found contacts in Nairobi, Kenya, who were willing to help ESPE in setting up a training programme that was to become a thorough 15-months' training. Experienced ESPE members (including myself) and some non-European paediatric endocrinologists have taken 1- to 2-month turns in tutoring. By now, 29 fellows from five African countries have been through the training, which I regard as highly successful.

ESPE is a democratic institution where each member has a vote at the Annual Business Meetings. One might therefore think that countries with many members would take all the important positions in ESPE. This has not been the case. A small country like Sweden has contributed many council members (including myself as chair of the Programme Organizing Committee for 6 years, the present Treasurer Olle Söder who is now ending his 6-year term of duty and the Secretary-Elect Lars Sävendahl). Swedish paediatric endocrinologists have organized one Annual Meeting and one Joint Meeting. ESPE awards have gone to several Swedes; The Andrea Prader Prize to myself, the ESPE Research Award to Kerstin Albertsson-Wikland, and the Outstanding Clinician Award to Otto Westphal.

The Joint Meeting in Stockholm in 1997 was a big challenge. The Local Organizing Committee included no honorary members, but only hard-working members of our own team, who did a wonderful job! By then, the Annual Meetings had grown to around one thousand participants, and a Joint Meeting was expected to draw up to 1,500 delegates. No suitable conference hall was available at that time in central Stockholm. But by combining a small conference centre, a former school, and large tents on the school yard (the latter for the poster exhibition) it worked! The Stockholm Joint Meeting might be remembered for its science, but also for the beautiful weather, the bright Nordic summer nights, and the excursion of the whole group, transported by seven old motor yachts to the fortress of Waxholm, in the Stockholm archipelago.

ESPE meetings have a tradition of being very social, with old and young participants enjoying not only science but also the company of each other. With the increase in delegate numbers to several thousands, it is no longer possible to arrange the 1-day excursion to make people meet in a relaxed atmosphere. But, as opposed to most other international conferences, setting up a dancing party has been an obligatory task for every local organizer, and I hope that this tradition will continue! Personally, I will continue coming to the annual meetings in yet a new city, to learn what is new in the field, take part in discussions, but also to meet my many international friends, old and young!

Personal Recollections

Sippell WG (ed): ESPE – The First 50 Years. A History of the European Society for Paediatric Endocrinology.
Basel, Karger, 2011, pp 111–114

Fulfilment and Fallibility: The Reflections of an ESPE Secretary (1997–2004)

Martin Savage, UK

Let me make it clear from the start that the 'fulfilment' refers to the satisfaction in the growth and development of ESPE and the 'fallibility' refers to the human weaknesses of the Secretary! Taking over as ESPE Secretary in 1997 was a daunting experience. I remember clearly the trip to Kiel in my Renault Espace, with all the seats except the driver's taken out, to visit my predecessor Wolfgang Sippell and transport the ESPE files back to London. Wolfgang was an admirable ESPE Secretary in every way. He had respected and upheld the traditions and high standards of the Society, while expanding the membership and clearly establishing ESPE as the leading international paediatric endocrinology society.

My abiding preoccupation was – am I up to this task? I think this was a natural concern, but looking back on the first years of my tenure as Secretary, it might have been more appropriate to ask myself – how can I build on Wolfgang's development of ESPE, rather than trying to keep things going as they were before. The next seven years were to prove challenging, enjoyable and revealing, not least of my own strengths and weaknesses.

The Secretariat

To take on the responsibilities of ESPE Secretary at the same time as running a paediatric endocrinology referral unit virtually single handed in central London initially presented a major challenge of organisation. I decided I could to it, but only with a significant contribution direct from ESPE to my own secretary's salary. This would allow her to devote sufficient time to Secretariat duties to keep the Society going. I needed to persuade the Treasurer, Sten Drop, that additional financial support, compared with past years, was necessary. Sten, an extremely wise and rather prudent financial administrator, in addition to his major scientific talents, needed some convincing. Eventually common sense prevailed.

With the Secretariat in place, the work really started. I was fortunate that Lorraine Greenwood, my own academic secretary, was an extraordinarily efficient and totally unflappable person, who enjoyed the work and in particular enjoyed coming to several ESPE meetings with her husband Mark to attend the ESPE stand. If Lorraine had not been so efficient, I would have realised sooner that to run a major scientific society, with all its demands and aspirations, with a single-handed Secretariat, sited in the office of a busy academic clinical paediatric endocrinologist, was an arrangement that could not endure permanently. A good management consultancy company would have seen this instantly; however, it took me a good three years to start embarking on a strategy to change this state of affairs. I will expand on this later.

Opening the Society to the Outside World
The 2000 Annual ESPE Meeting in Brussels marked a pivotal milestone in the development of the Society. The criteria of eligibility for application for ESPE membership, as stated in the Constitution, were clearly defined and consisted of presentations at previous Annual Meetings and residency in a 'European or Mediterranean' country. Many ESPE members were happy with this situation, but in 2000, I was presented with a particular challenge. For the first time, a doctor from outside the designated geographical region approached me about applying for ESPE membership. Dr Mariam Razzaghy-Azar from Teheran had faithfully attended and contributed to ESPE meetings for many years. She saw the potential benefits of being a member of the Society and was keen to apply. Council scrutinized and approved her application, but also recognised that to elect her would constitute a 'test case'.

Now I will describe the first instance of human fallibility. Her application was duly processed and her name appeared on the list of members for election, usually accepted with a show of hands, which I presented at the Annual Business Meeting in Brussels. The problem was that I had forgotten that Mariam's name and country of origin appeared on the list. Had I remembered, I would have made reference to this and described her potential election as a departure from normal practice and even an exception to the Constitution. However, expecting everything to go through as in previous years, I was taken aback and somewhat embarrassed when a senior ESPE member quite correctly put up his hand and pointed out that to elect a doctor from Iran would contravene the terms of the Constitution.

Sometimes, one has to think on one's feet and I was fortunate that the ESPE membership is unfailingly generous, tolerant, friendly and forward-looking. Although Mariam could not be elected that year, an opportunity had presented itself to sow the seeds of opening the Society beyond the existing geographical boundaries – but of course the Constitution would need changing to permit this. I asked for a show of hands to support the principle of removing these boundaries with the possibility of opening the Society to the rest of the world. There was a clear majority who supported this idea in an unofficial vote, which allowed changes to be made and me to regain a little personal pride!

The next challenge was to change the Constitution, which was in fact achieved several times during the next few years. With the geographical restrictions removed, Mariam Razzaghy-Azar became the first 'non-European' ESPE member. Since then, the other criteria of eligibility have been modified and ESPE has become a truly global Society with members from the USA, the Middle East, Australia, South America and the Far East.

Professional Management for ESPE

Another defining moment for me as Secretary came at the end of the very successful Joint Lawson Wilkins-ESPE meeting in Montreal in 2001. As other ESPE Secretaries will readily testify, the Annual Meeting is a satisfying but exhausting experience. This was particularly true for the Montreal Meeting. The local organising Committee had generously accommodated me in a suite at the Queen Elizabeth Congress Hotel and I had booked my flight back home 48 hours after the end of the meeting, having anticipated a certain amount of post-meeting administrative work. This work in fact took me 12 solid hours to complete and after I had dictated the minutes of the sixth committee meeting, I was convinced that this was work best suited to an efficient administrative company and not to a harassed endocrinologist with an increasingly fragile memory.

My conviction was as always supported in principle by Council and we went on to form a Strategic Management Committee, chaired by Stephen Shalet, with the aim of addressing the issue of out-sourcing the ESPE Secretariat. We interviewed candidate companies for this contract and duly appointed BioScientifica, a UK company based in Bristol with particular experience of supporting scientific societies.

While on the subject of out-sourcing, I must get another issue 'off my chest'. The year 2000 also marked the advent of the electronic world in terms of abstract submission and organisation of the scientific programme. Marc Maes, the excellent ESPE President in 2000, quite rightly felt that a change of conference organising company should be considered for future Annual Meetings. A small working group was formed to consider candidates for this contract. I was wisely advised not to make a commitment for more than one year and we interviewed a number of companies to run the electronic abstract submission process for the 2001 meeting in Madrid.

With the best intentions, we made the wrong choice! A group of doctors is not the best committee to choose a commercial organisation. I have always felt badly because the organisation of the meeting in Madrid was made infinitely more difficult for the President, Jesús Argente and his wife Julie. There is no question that Jesús and Julie suffered from our lack of insight. Despite this, the Madrid meeting was an outstanding success. Professionals should choose professionals. This was another sign that the organisation of ESPE was becoming too challenging and too important to be left in the hands of doctors.

Humble Pie and Fulfilment

Hubris can be the product of success. By 2003, ESPE was in a strong position. Now acknowledged as the leading paediatric endocrinology society, each successive meeting had attracted record attendance and the quality of the scientific programme was recognised to be of considerable scientific and educational value. The meetings such as those in Florence, Brussels, Madrid and Basel had brought me great personal satisfaction. ESPE seemed to be on the crest of a wave. What could go wrong?

The Constitution had been redrafted and a new structure of committees was in place with a democratic system of elections to Council. The procedure for the election of the new Secretary was clear and an excellent candidate, Francesco Chiarelli from Chieti applied. The procedure should have been straight forward. For some reason, which I never really understood, an opinion within the Society was gaining strength that there should be two candidates – to give a more democratic election. Very unwisely, I listened to the voices proposing this course of action and even encouraged an alternative candidate to consider applying. This was a major error of judgement and directly insulting to Franco Chiarelli and his Italian supporters. It was also confusing and disrespectful to the potential alternative candidate. It took a phone call to me from my mentor Jean-Louis Chaussain in Paris informing me that a mass resignation of Italian ESPE members was imminent to make me see sense.

Hubris had clouded my judgement. This was not my finest hour! I was delighted that a successor as talented and committed as Franco was duly elected as the next ESPE Secretary. He generously refers to me as his mentor, but it is his humility and qualities as a listener that shine through. I find fulfilment in the true leadership he has shown together with a rare ability to combine confidence with service. The Society has thrived at an even greater pace. Applications for membership from all over the world are pouring in and ESPE is truly seen as a beacon of scientific and educational excellence. We are in a very strong position.

Last Thoughts

It was an enormous privilege to lead an organisation such as ESPE. I made many friends and received enormous support. On the positive side, the ESPE Research Unit and the ESPE Corporate Liaison Board were created and the Secretariat was successfully outsourced to a professional management company. The Constitution was 'modernised' and new committee structures were put in place.

I have to say, I enjoyed every, or almost every, moment of the seven years. Leadership presents unique and sometimes unexpected challenges. Confidence and humility should occupy juxtapositions – but beware of the hubris!

Personal Recollections

Sippell WG (ed): ESPE – The First 50 Years. A History of the European Society for Paediatric Endocrinology.
Basel, Karger, 2011, pp 115–118

Happy Birthday to ESPE, a Fine Example of European Integration

Wolfgang G. Sippell, Germany

I started my endocrinology lab research as a young post-doc under Professor Dieter Knorr in the cold, humid basement of the old Hauner-Kinderspital of Munich University, trying to isolate and measure multiple steroids from very small blood samples. When I had obtained the first plausible results with my new method, I was told that *the* place to present such data was the ESPE meeting, taking place that year (1975) in Berlin. Since I was late, all the ESPE members in our group, Dieter Knorr, Otfrid Butenandt and Frank Bidlingmaier, had already invited a guest. I therefore had to ask the President, Professor Hans Helge, who readily accepted my abstract.

I was very impressed by the well-organised meeting, the very friendly atmosphere among the 200 or so participants and the amount of time allowed for discussing the results presented. Everybody seemed to know everybody. It was also an excellent opportunity to see and meet, for the first time, the senior colleagues from the other major research groups in West Germany, such as Jürgen Bierich, Walter Teller, Dieter Schönberg, Werner Blunck, Bruno Weber and others.

From then on I attended almost every ESPE meeting, and it was the yearly highlight of my professional and scientific life. Most German colleagues felt the same and for many years were convinced that there was no need for a separate German paediatric endocrinology group, since ESPE meetings with their comprehensive programmes, scientific exchange and social contacts met all our expectations.

However, it was not easy to become an ESPE member in those days and even if somebody was scientifically active and had already presented twice at ESPE meetings, the application, backed by two senior ESPE members, still had to 'lie on the table' for at least 1 year until Council proposed the author as a new member for individual election at the next business meeting. Colleagues who were not involved in research or who were not invited as a guest by an ESPE member could not participate at ESPE meetings.

For this reason, during the lovely boat cruise on Lago Maggiore at the 1980 Bergamo meeting, a group of German ESPE members agreed informally to found a German Working Group for Paediatric Endocrinology with relatively open access, in order to be able to hold an annual German meeting which was separate from the established German paediatric and endocrinology congresses, and focussed primarily on the presentation and discussion of joint studies. Its first chairman ('speaker') was Werner Blunck, who was succeeded by Michael Ranke.

As an ESPE Council member from 1981 to 1984, I remember the preparation and realisation of the first ESPE meeting behind the Iron Curtain as a particular highlight. It was held in 1983 in Budapest under the excellent presidency of Feri Péter, the founder of paediatric endocrinology in Hungary. For the first time, the West German participants were able to meet their East German colleagues who, with the exception of a few party members, were not allowed to travel to the ESPE meetings in Western Europe. This was a wonderful opportunity. The meeting venue, a beautiful, old city palace, was guarded by a police officer sitting at the entrance and checking our passports, resulting in an excellent attendance rate at the scientific sessions since nobody dared to sneak out for sightseeing or shopping in between.

Feri Péter became a very good and trusted friend who, without hesitation and at personal risk to himself and his wife, helped my East German god-son to escape across the Hungarian-Yugoslav border to the West in the summer of 1989 – at that time nobody could imagine that the Iron Curtain would fall just a few months later!

Another project which would never have been realised without ESPE was a study conceived during the 1984 annual meeting in Heidelberg as I sat together with our one-time Secretary Al Aynsley-Green over a tasty glass of Palatinate wine. I was shocked to hear from Al that, in order to avoid postoperative ventilatory depression, newborn babies in the UK, the Commonwealth countries and the USA were still undergoing surgery with only nitrous oxide and curare used as regular 'shallow' anaesthesia, the so-called 'Liverpool method'. In contrast, in continental Europe Fentanyl (a powerful analgesic) had already been in use for many years in anaesthesia, even for premature babies. With his gifted MD candidate, Kanwal Anand, Al designed and carried out a small randomised trial in which we measured all relevant adrenal stress hormones and metabolites longitudinally in microlitre amounts of plasma from preterm babies undergoing standardised Botalli duct surgery. The results showed huge, abnormal increases in adrenal hormones and glucose reflecting stress and pain, as well as significant postoperative complications in the non-Fentanyl group. Our Lancet paper [1] precipitated a heated public debate in the UK but quickly led to a strict ban of the Liverpool method around the world – not least thanks to ESPE!

My second term in Council, 1991–1997, the last 5 years of which as Secretary, was a considerable challenge in terms of extra work and responsibilities but it also brought lots of pleasure and rewarding personal relationships with many friends, both within and outside ESPE. Planning the programmes of the two Joint meetings in San Francisco 1993 and in Stockholm 1997 particularly served to strengthen the friendly relations with our colleagues in the North American LWPES as well as with those in the cooperating societies around the world, SLEP, APPES and JSPE.

During this time the necessity to establish a permanent secretariat to cope with the affairs of the rapidly growing Society was becoming increasingly clear. The ever increasing work of English correspondence, minutes of Council meetings and the increasing number of committees would not have been manageable at all without the expert help and efficient support of Joanna Voerste, my secretarial assistant for so many years.

One of my main goals during my time as Secretary was to open ESPE's doors towards Eastern Europe, where colleagues were now no longer restricted in their scientific contacts and travel to western Europe. The only obstacle for them now was lack of money. We were successful in convincing pharmaceutical companies, particularly those which produced recombinant human growth hormone, to fund new longer term educational ESPE programmes set up especially for young colleagues from eastern European countries, where training in paediatric endocrinology, including diabetes, was not yet adequate. Among my personally most satisfying achievements as ESPE Secretary were the establishment of the Clinical Fellowship, supported by Serono, in 1992 and of the Winter School, supported by Ferring, which was first held in 1994.

Last but not least and looking back, my fondest memories related to ESPE are the sailing trips from Kiel to the annual meetings in Copenhagen (3 days), Stockholm (6 days), Rotterdam (6 days) and, after my retirement, to Helsinki (12 days) and, of course, back home again, usually by a slightly different route. ESPE friends and young colleagues from my group in Kiel often acted as crew, which was always enjoyable, even if one had to rehearse the ESPE presentation during the hours off duty from the tiller. Luckily we never ran into major weather or technical problems, always arriving ahead of time to a comfortable guest harbour near the meeting venue, thus saving me the cost of an expensive hotel room! I enjoyed being able to offer a drink on board to my Council friends in Stockholm's Vaasa harbour, thanking them at the end of my time as secretary, and to my respected senior ESPE friend Henk Visser and his wife Margaret in Rotterdam's historic Veerhaven harbour, thanking him for his dedicated work, without which ESPE would not have survived its perinatal period. Incidentally, Henk was also an ESPE pioneer in nautical terms, having sailed the long stretch from Rotterdam to Helsinki and back on the occasion of the first Helsinki meeting in 1982.

Finally, I can only concur with my fellow contributors and, I feel sure, with the majority of ESPE members today, that in its 50th year ESPE is still, and will hopefully continue to be, much more than an excellent sounding board for international science: it offers lasting good personal relations and friendship across both borders and generations.

Reference

1 Anand KJS, Sippell WG, Aynsley-Green A: Randomised trial of Fentanyl anaesthesia in preterm babies undergoing surgery: effects on the stress response. Lancet 1987;i:243–248.

Personal Recollections

'Back to the Vikings': Paediatric Endocrinology in Denmark

Niels E. Skakkebaek and Knud W. Kastrup, Denmark

The cradle of Danish paediatric endocrinology stood at the Queen Louise Children's Hospital in Copenhagen where Henning Andersen established an endocrine clinic in 1950. He served as a visiting fellow at Johns Hopkins with Lawson Wilkins in 1952 and was appointed in 1964 to the chair at the Children's Hospital, Fuglebakken, to which he moved the paediatric endocrine activities.

In 1971, Henning Andersen was appointed professor of Paediatrics at the University of Copenhagen. He retired in 1977 and passed away in 1978.

After Henning Andersen moved to Fuglebakken (1964), the endocrine clinic became a national referral centre and attracted a number of paediatricians, being the only place in Denmark where special training in this field could be obtained. Both the clinic, and the laboratory where Knud W. Kastrup had established the first somatomedin assays in Denmark, moved to Hvidovre Hospital after the closure of the Children's Hospital Fuglebakken in 1983. From there the endocrine clinic was transferred to Rigshospitalet in 1990 and embedded into the University Department of Growth and Reproduction, established by Niels E. Skakkebaek in the same year.

Henning Andersen was instrumental in creating The Nordic Grant for the Study of Growth, succeeded by the ESPE Research Fellowship. His name is also attached to the Henning Andersen Prize, which was instituted in 1988 in memory of his personal importance and interest for ESPE and paediatric endocrinology in general.

The history of the manufacture of growth hormone goes back to 1947 when the first studies of the effect of growth hormone in mice were published. Henning Andersen contacted H.C. Hagedorn at Nordisk Insulinlaboratorium in 1966 and encouraged this institution to initiate the production of human pituitary growth hormone, a production which is still ongoing, now in the form of biosynthetic GH at Novo-Nordisk.

Dr. Erik Thamdrup was a very close collaborator of Henning Andersen, and his thesis 'Precocious Sexual Development' in 1961 was published as a highly cited monograph. Dr. Thamdrup was a lifelong member of ESPE and member of the paediatric endocrine team as a consultant at the endocrine clinic.

Henning Andersen became a close friend of Lawson Wilkins, who visited Copenhagen on several occasions. Henning Andersen's son Johannes has given a vivid description of Dr. Wilkins' personality and the special relations he had with Henning Andersen and his family. They shared some characteristic personal traits and sense of humour. According to Henning Andersen, Lawson Wilkins claimed that he could trace his family back to the Vikings and often saluted them by proposing a toast. Especially, he saluted one great, great, great grandmother who was overwhelmed by a Viking without much resistance, leading him to believe that he was related to Harald Bluetooth, the first Danish king to be christened.

The Copenhagen team organized the 1988 ESPE meeting. In contrast to the current situation, the ESPE meetings of that time were meetings for members and their guests only. Therefore, there was a special spirit of 'paediatric endocrinology academia' at the meetings during these early years of the society. It was quite difficult to become an ESPE member at that time and far from all who wanted to participate were admitted. In this respect, the local organizing committee had to handle a very difficult situation. A couple of weeks before the meeting in 1988, the President was contacted by one of the major pharmaceutical companies, which had sponsored the meeting and asked whether 25 paediatricians (not ESPE members) could be registered. The request was declined according to the rules. In spite of this the same 25 persons came to the registration desk shortly before the opening of the meeting. The secretaries at the registration desk did not know what to do. An ‹emergency council meeting› was held on the spot, and it was decided that the group of doctors, who most likely were ‹medical tourists› without a genuine interest in paediatric endocrinology, could not be accepted as participants. In spite of this strict policy there were approximately 300 registered and for the first time parallel sessions were held.

Hosting the ESPE meeting was a great stimulus for paediatric endocrinology in Copenhagen. It might even have been of importance for establishing the University Department of Growth and Reproduction, which was inaugurated at Rigshospitalet in 1990. The department is unique, being an independent institution with its own administration and budget and focus on paediatric endocrinology as well as on male reproduction. The reproductive part of the activities was a continuation of an existing laboratory of Reproductive Biology at Rigshospitalet, which Niels Skakkebaek had coordinated since the 1970s. The paediatric part included the endocrine clinic and laboratory which were transferred to Rigshospitalet from Hvidovre Hospital. During the past 20 years, the staff of the Department of Growth and Reproduction has grown from 17 persons to more than 80 today. Since 2006, Anders Juul has been chairman of the department, which in 2010 was awarded a prize from the Capital Region of Copenhagen as a Center of International Excellence. The annual activities include

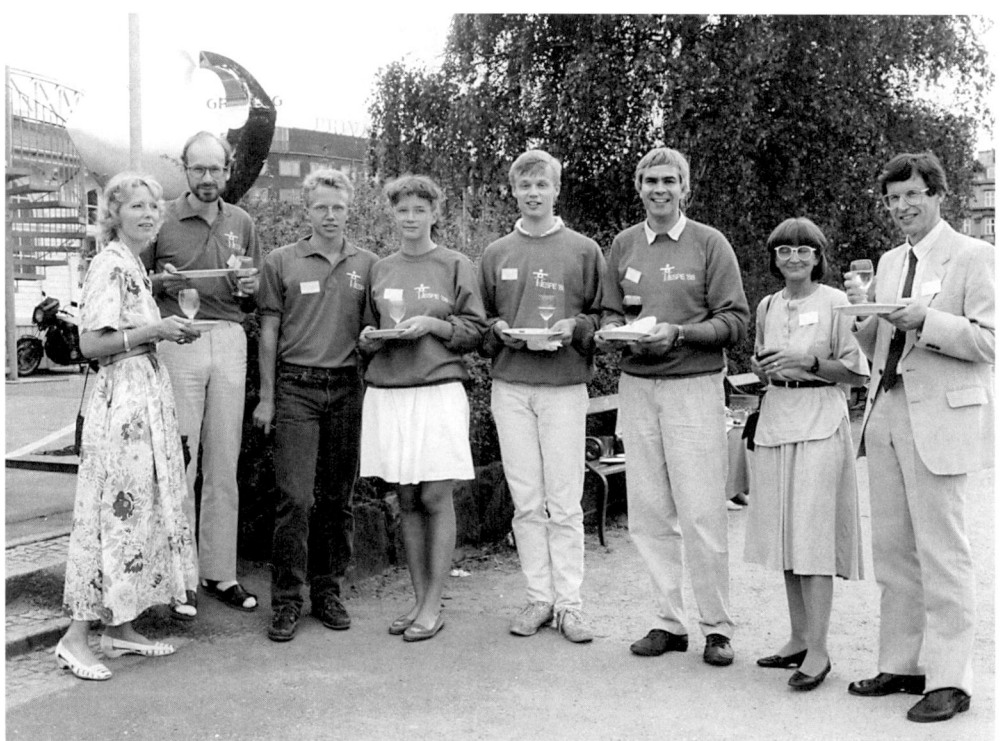

The President of the 1988 ESPE Meeting in Stockholm and his team.

more than 10,000 patient visits in the outpatient clinic, and 40–50 research papers, besides several doctoral theses each year. (Please see www.reproduction.dk for more information.)

ESPE from a Personal and Finnish Perspective

Raimo Voutilainen, Finland

ESPE Annual and Related Meetings

My personal contact with ESPE started in 1982 when the 21st Annual Meeting was arranged in Helsinki with Professor Jaakko Perheentupa as the president. He had attended ESPE Annual Meetings since the Malmö meeting (Sweden) in 1969. My modest role in the Helsinki 1982 meeting was to work as a voluntary 'slide boy' taking care and showing the slides of speakers during oral sessions. In that meeting I did not have any scientific presentation of my own. The second Annual ESPE Meeting I attended was in Budapest 1983. My first abstract in any international scientific meeting dealing with growth in Cushing's syndrome was not a great success: it was in the category 'Read by title'. The third annual meeting I attended was in Heidelberg 1984. There was some progress from the previous year: I had my first oral presentation in any international meeting. The topic of the abstract was the effect of ACTH treatment on serum adrenal androgen concentrations in infants with infantile spasms. The work showed that ACTH increases adrenal androgen production already in infancy and suggested that no specific adrenal androgen-stimulating hormone is needed. At that time there was an assumption (presented even in many textbooks) that a specific pituitary adrenal androgen-stimulating hormone exists. Later experimental and clinical research have confirmed that ACTH is needed for adrenal androgen production in normal adrenals, and no other specific adrenal androgen-stimulating hormone has been found or is needed.

In 1985–1986 I could not attend the ESPE meetings due to my postdoctoral training abroad, lack of new scientific data to be presented, and the poor funding situation. I did my postdoctoral training in Walter Miller's laboratory in San Francisco in 1985–1986. At that time, ESPE did not (to my knowledge) have any research fellowships or other awards to support foreign training. Thus, my fellowship was not linked to ESPE, but that period much influenced my later contacts and activities in

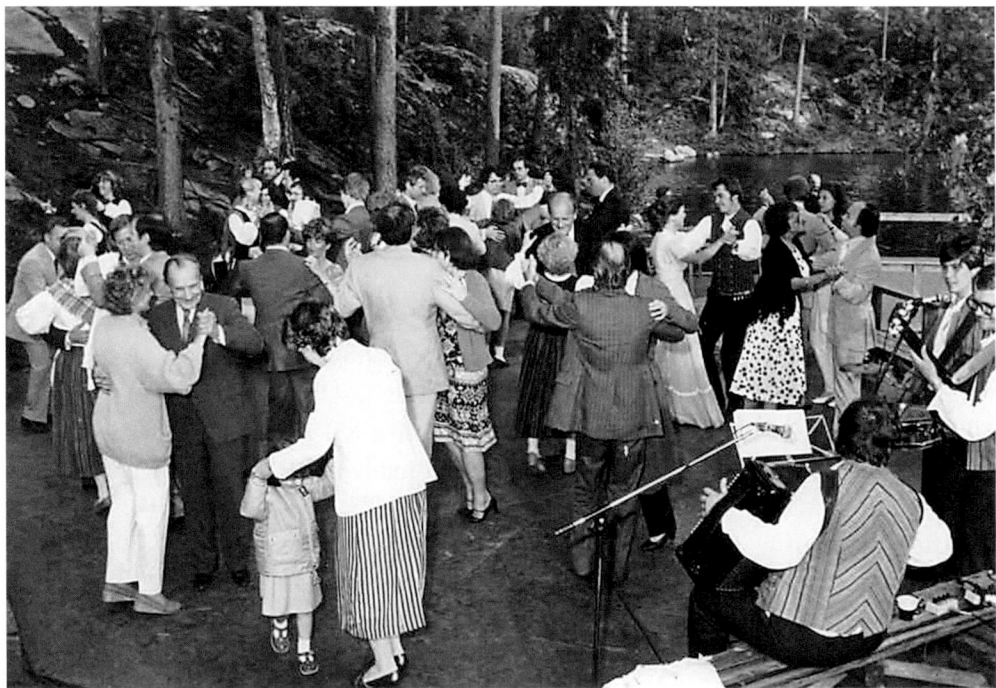

A dancing event outdoors at the 1982 ESPE meeting in Helsinki. The dancing pair at the right is Ruth Illig and Charles Brook.

ESPE. Although my postdoctoral fellowship was an economically tough time (low level Finnish funding during a period of very strong US dollar), it was a scientifically productive and rewarding time. The human cDNAs for the key steroidogenic genes (P450scc, P450c21 and P450c17) were just cloned in Walter Miller's laboratory when I started there. I had an excellent opportunity to use these cDNAs for studying the expression of those genes in human foetal adrenal and gonadal samples, and also in human adult ovarian granulosa cells obtained from women undergoing in vitro fertilization. The success and productivity of my post-doctoral period was much based on collaboration with and human tissue material supplied by Juha Tapanainen, a Finnish post-doc working partly at the same time at the Department of Obstetrics, Gynecology and Reproductive Sciences of the same campus. Juha provided me with human foetal testicular and ovarian samples he had collected and taught me how to culture ovarian granulosa cells. His contribution was quite essential, I owe him a lot. At that time I also met Juha's wife, Päivi Tapanainen, for the first time, a future paediatric endocrinologist and an active ESPE member, who was taking her first scientific steps in the San Francisco Pediatric Endocrine Unit under Selna Kaplan's supervision. I want to acknowledge and thank Walter Miller for my 2-year post-doctoral period in his research group. He was an excellent and enthusiastic teacher in both molecular biology and scientific writing. Although his research group was small at that time,

I was lucky to be there at an optimal time having the privilege to apply the molecular biological tools the group had just developed. Walter also allowed me to study those topics I was personally interested in. During my post-doctoral period in San Francisco, I also had the opportunity to follow the weekly clinical paediatric endocrine patient meetings and thus also became clinically trained. The lively discussions and arguments with many real experts in paediatric endocrinology (Selna Kaplan, Melvin Gumbach, Felix Conte, Stephen Rosenthal among others) were enjoyable and really educational.

I want to emphasize Walter Miller's role as a trainer of many other European postdoctoral fellows in his laboratory. After my visit he hosted for instance Yves Morel from France, Wiebke Arlt from Germany (currently in UK) and Christa Flück from Switzerland. All these persons have later been active ESPE members or speakers in ESPE meetings. Walter himself has also attended many ESPE meetings, giving excellent presentations.

After completing my post-doctoral training I have attended all ESPE Annual Meetings since 1987. Personally, I consider three of these meetings most memorable (1989, 2002, 2007). In 1989, the annual meeting was a joint meeting with LWPES in Jerusalem, Israel. The abstract I had submitted was selected as the winner of the Henning Andersen Prize. I can remember well the session chaired by the president of that meeting, Zvi Laron. The Madrid ESPE meeting in 2002 was another important meeting for personal and national reasons. We applied and won the responsibility for arranging the 2007 annual meeting. After many years' preparation, the 26th Annual ESPE Meeting in Helsinki was naturally the most demanding and memorable ESPE meeting personally. I want to express my gratitude to the Finnish Paediatric Endocrine Society, the Local Organising Committee, and Congrex for their contribution and support in the meeting arrangements. Especially Päivi Miettinen and Timo Otonkoski were key persons in the practical arrangements of the meeting, and Tiina Laine took care of the ESPE Summer School; thanks to them once more.

ESPE Council and Committees

I had the opportunity to work as a member of the ESPE Council in 1995–1998. Wolfgang Sippell and Martin Savage lead the council work during that time period as Secretaries of the society. Both of them created an efficient and pleasant atmosphere for the council work, with their own personalities. Typical for Wolfgang was his German punctuality. On the basis of common scientific interests and personal contacts in ESPE, we collaborated with each other later. This led to a joint publication on adrenocortical function in premature newborns. Martin Savage, a real British gentleman, impressed among other things with his excellent French language. From the other council members I remember especially Stephen Shalet's significant and active contribution to council work. From 2005 to 2007, I had the pleasure to work in the council for a second time as the president elect and president when preparing for the 2007 annual meeting to be held in Helsinki. Francesco Chiarelli led the council with his enthusiastic and firm control. I thank him very much for his strong support in the preparation for the ESPE 2007 meeting. Ze'ev Hochberg chaired the Programme Organising Committee between 2004 and 2007. His energy and efforts to the highest possible quality of the meeting programmes were admirable. Although he often had strong opinions of his own, he accepted well-grounded suggestions to the programme from the local organisers, which we much appreciated.

I had the opportunity to chair the ESPE Sabbatical Leave Committee in 2008–2010, after serving some years as an ordinary member of the committee during the chairmanship of Marc Maes. Eli Lilly has supported the programme since 1993, and I had also received support from the programme in 1996 for my sabbatical leave in Cambridge, UK. Lilly had changed its support policy in 2008, which meant that a grant application had to be sent to the Lilly Grant Office every year for the ESPE Sabbatical Leave Programme. This process increased the work load of the committee and made the support for the programme difficult to predict and guarantee. Jan-Maarten Wit and Paolo Beck-Beccoz have served as efficient committee members evaluating the grant applications. Thanks to them and to Lilly for the support of the programme for many years.

Finnish ESPE Prize and Award Winners
Hans Åkerblom received the Andrea Prader Prize in 1998 and Mikael Knip the ESPE Research Award in 2006 for their long-term diabetes studies. Jaakko Perheentupa was acknowledged by the Outstanding Clinician Award in 2002. To my knowledge, he was asked several times to submit documents for the nomination of Andrea Prader Prize, but he as a modest man wrongly considered himself unqualified for that prize. His merits as a researcher, teacher and clinician in paediatric endocrinology are remarkable. He is the founder of paediatric endocrinology in Finland and has trained a whole generation of paediatric endocrinologists for the country. Leo Dunkel received the ESPE Research award in 2008; his research interests have been especially in puberty and in its disorders. Two Finns have received the ESPE Young Investigator Award based on their high quality publications. Päivi Miettinen received it in 1997 and Taneli Raivio in 2004. Three Finns have won the Henning Andersen Prizes. I had the honour to be the first in 1989 when I presented my abstract in the ESPE/LWPES Joint Meeting. Hanna Huopio received the Henning Andersen Prize in 1998 and Timo Otonkoski in 2003. Their abstracts dealt with congenital hyperinsulinism and the respective data have later been published in highly appreciated scientific journals. Many of the current Finnish paediatric endocrinologists have also received support from the ESPE Research Fellowship Programme, allowing research work in foreign research centres. Päivi Tapanainen, Leo Dunkel, Päivi Miettinen, Jarmo Jääskeläinen and Outi Mäkitie have since been supported by the full research fellowships of this programme.

ESPE Facts

Annual ESPE Meetings

Overview of the Annual ESPE Meetings

Date	Venue	President
1962	Zurich, Switzerland	Andrea Prader
1963	Groningen, Netherlands	Hendrick K.A. Visser
1964	Hamburg, Germany	Jürgen R. Bierich
1965	Copenhagen, Denmark	Henning J. Andersen
1966	Glasgow, UK	William Hamilton
1967	Haifa, Israel	Zvi Laron
1968	Vienna, Austria	Walter Swoboda
1969	Malmö, Sweden	Carl G. Bergstrand
1970	Lyon, France	René François
1971	Zurich, Switzerland	José M. Frances / Andrea Prader
1972	Louvain, Belgium	Paul Malvaux
1973	Bergen, Norway	Dagfinn Aarskog
1974	Paris, France	Pierre Royer
1975	Berlin, Germany	Hans Helge
1976	Rotterdam, Netherlands	Hendrick K.A. Visser
1977	Cambridge, UK	Charles G.D. Brook
1978	Athens, Greece	Catherine Dacou-Voutetakis
1979	Ulm, Germany	Walter Teller
1980	Bergamo, Italy	Giuseppe Chiumello
1981	* Geneva, Switzerland	Pierre C. Sizonenko
1982	Helsinki, Finland	Jaakko Perheentupa
1983	Budapest, Hungary	Ferenc Péter
1984	Heidelberg, Germany	Dieter Schönberg
1985	* Baltimore, USA	Raphael Rappaport
1986	Zurich, Switzerland	Ruth Illig

Date	Venue	President
1987	Toulouse, France	Pierre Rochiccioli
1988	Copenhagen, Denmark	Niels Skakkebaek
1989	* Jerusalem, Israel	Zvi Laron
1990	Vienna, Austria	Herwig Frisch
1991	Berlin, Germany	Volker Hesse
1992	Zaragoza, Spain	Angel Ferrández Longás
1993	* San Francisco, USA	Ieuan A. Hughes
1994	Maastricht, Netherlands	J. Leo Van den Brande
1995	Edinburgh, UK	Albert Aynsley-Green
1996	Montpellier, France	Charles Sultan
1997	* Stockholm, Sweden	Martin Ritzén
1998	Florence, Italy	Giorgio Giovannelli
1999	Warsaw, Poland	Thomasz E. Romer
2000	Brussels, Belgium	Marc Maes
2001	* Montreal, Canada	Guy Van Vliet / Harvey Guyda
2002	Madrid, Spain	Jesús Argente
2003	Ljubljana, Slovenia	Ciril Krzisnik
2004	Basel, Switzerland	Ze'ev Hochberg
2005	* Lyon, France	Yves Morel
2006	Rotterdam, Netherlands	Stenvert L.S. Drop
2007	Helsinki, Finland	Raimo Voutilainen
2008	Istanbul, Turkey	Atilla Büyükgebiz
2009	* New York, USA	Francesco Chiarelli
2010	Prague, Czech Republic	Jan Lebl
2011	Glasgow, UK	Chris Kelnar

* Joint Meeting with the Lawson Wilkins Pediatric Endocrine Society (LWPES, changed name to Pediatric Endocrine Society (PES) recently) of North America, from 1997 in collaboration with the Australasian Paediatric Endocrine Group (APEG), the Japanese Society for Pediatric Endocrinology (JSPE) and the Sociedad Latino-Americana de Endocrinologia Pediatrica (SLEP); since 2005 also with the Asia Pacific Endocrine Society (APPES).

Annual ESPE Meetings 1962–2011

1962 Zurich	1st Meeting
Date:	8th to 10th July
Venue:	Kinderspital (Children's Hospital), University of Zurich, Switzerland
President:	Andrea Prader (CH)
Participants (n):	32
Abstracts (n):	none

Scientific programme:

10 short (10–15 min) presentations followed by extensive (30–45 min) free discussions about: Steroid purification from urine by paper chromatography (Bush system); The use of anabolic steroids in dwarfism: The metabolic effects of human growth hormone, its extraction from human pituitaries, antibody formation, etc. (A. Prader); Adrenal diseases; sexual precocity; Parathyroids and rickets.

Social programme:

Boat trip on Lake Zurich, dinner in Horgen.

Sponsors: None

1963 Groningen	2nd Annual Meeting, 'European Paediatric Endocrinology Club'
Date:	5th to 8th May
Venue:	Lecture Room, Department of Paediatrics, University Hospital Groningen, The Netherlands
President:	Hendrick K.A. Visser (NL)
Participants (n):	50 active, 11 accompanying persons
Abstracts (n):	33, published in Acta Endocrinol 1964;45(suppl 89):S9–S43

Scientific programme:

Diagnostic methods (measurement of HGH in plasma, evaluation of pituitary-adrenal and pituitary-thyroid function); Clinical problems (e.g. first report by H.K.A. Visser on a familiar salt-losing syndrome due to deficient 18-hydroxylation, later known as the Visser-Cost syndrome).

Social programme:
Welcome by the University's Rector Magnificus; Dinner at National Coach Museum, Leek; Cocktail and dinner at Clubhuis, Paterswolde; Full day bus excursion, including a visit to the bulb fields and lunch at Keukenhof. – Ladies: excursion to North Friesland (Menkemaborgh castle); Walking tour of old Groningen.

Sponsors: Organon N.V. (Oss, The Netherlands), Ciba N.V. (Basel, Switzerland), Nutricia N.V. (Zoetermeer, The Netherlands).

1964 Hamburg	3rd Annual Meeting, 'European Paediatric Endocrinology Club'
Date:	19th to 22nd April
Venue:	Lecture Hall, Paediatric Department, University Hospital Eppendorf, Hamburg, West Germany
President:	Jürgen R. Bierich (D)
Secretary:	H.K.A. Visser (NL)
Council:	A. Prader (CH), Henning Andersen (DK), William Hamilton (UK), René François (F)
Participants (n):	55 active, 15 accompanying persons
Abstracts (n):	35, published in Acta Endocrinol 1965;49(suppl 101):S7–S48

Scientific programme:
40 presentations of 10, 15 or 20 min followed by discussions of 10–25 min: Precocious puberty; Delayed puberty/lack of puberty; Undescended testes; Physiology and pathology of the adrenal glandps; Thyroid and parathyroids; Growth disturbances (e.g., first presentation of 'a new method for the evaluation of skeletal maturity' by J.M. Tanner – the TW2 method).

Social programme:
Welcome at clubhouse Norddeutscher Regattaverein; Dinner at Hamburger and Germania Ruderclub; Boat trip on the river Elbe including a visit to the harbour, lunch at a riverside village and tea at the Landungsbrücken Restaurant. – Ladies: Sightseeing tour Hamburg (Kunst- und Gewerbemuseum, Ernst-Barlach-Haus, Jenisch-Haus).

Sponsors: Ciba AG, N.V. Organon, Schering AG (Berlin)

1965 Copenhagen	4th Annual Meeting, 'European Paediatric Endocrinology Club' → ESPE
Date:	8th to 11th August
Venue:	Steno Memorial Hospital, Gentofte (Copenhagen), Denmark
President:	Henning J. Andersen (DK)
Secretary + Treasurer:	H.K.A. Visser (NL)
Council:	A. Prader (CH), J.R. Bierich (D), W. Hamilton (UK), R. François (F)
Participants (n):	49 active (19 members, 30 guests), 23 accompanying persons
Abstracts (n):	30
	The President informed participants 'that abstracts containing facts rather than promises will generally be preferred'. Publication in *Acta Endocrinologica* was planned but 'unfortunately' (Secretary's newsletter) it did not happen.

Scientific programme:

Two full days with plenary sessions, each consisting of 15 papers of 10-15 min, each followed by discussion of 5–10 min.

Growth and growth hormone determination; Urinary testosterone, cortisol excretion rates in health and disease; Insulin tolerance test, insulin excretion, glucosuria due to anabolics; Thyroxine and binding proteins; XO/XY syndrome; Prader-Willi syndrome; Adrenal insufficiency.

Social programme:

Reception at Domus Medica; Dinner at Langeliniepavillonen; Reception at Town Hall; Full day bus excursion to North Sealand: visit to the exhibition of modern art at Lousiana Museum and to Hamlet's Castle Kronborg at Helsingoer. – Ladies: Danish handicraft tour; Guided city tour (including 'a peep into Danish cooking mysteries').

Sponsors:	Alfred Benzon AS, Ferrosan AS, Nestle Nordisk AS, Nordisk Droge- og Kemikalieforretning AS, Nordisk Insulin Laboratorium, N.V. Organon, Upjohn International Inc., Winthrop Medicinalkompagni AS.

1966 Glasgow	5th Annual Meeting, ESPE
Date:	4th to 7th September
Venue:	Royal Hospital for Sick Children, Glasgow, UK
President:	William Hamilton (UK)
Secretary + Treasurer:	H.K.A. Visser (NL)
Council:	A. Prader (CH), J. Bierich (D), H. Andersen (DK), R. François (F)
Participants (n):	70 active (20 members, 50 guests), 15 accompanying persons
Abstracts (n):	33, not published (Board of *Pediatric Research* refused)

Scientific programme:

Two full days with 19 and 14 papers, respectively, each 10 min, followed by discussion. Growth hormone: immuno-assay techniques, nocturnal secretion, materno-foetal relationships, Turner's syndrome; Adrenal hyperplasia, steroid excretion patterns, hypoaldosteronism; Gonadal dysgenesis in twins; Congenital hypoparathyroidism, thyrocalcitonin, vitamin D-resistant rickets; Body composition during refeeding; Anti-androgen effects.

Social programme:

Reception at University College Club; Sherry reception by the Royal College of Physicians and Surgeons; Annual Dinner by the University Court at Randolph Hall; Full day tour around lochs of Central Scotland, evening: optional visit to Edinburgh Music Festival. – Ladies: Visit to Glasgow Cathedral, lunch in town with mannequin parade; Drive to Loch Lomond, Glen Fruin and Helensburgh (lunch), visit to tonsorial artist.

Sponsors:	William R. Warner & Co., Organon Laboratories, Ames Company, Pharmethicals, Upjohn, Hoechst, John Wyeth & Brother, Ciba Laboratories, Glaxo Laboratories, Lederle Laboratories, G.D. Searle & Co.

1967 Haifa	6th Annual Meeting, ESPE
Date:	19th to 24th March
Venue:	Ben Dori Recreation Home, Mt. Carmel, Haifa, Israel
President:	Zvi Laron (IL)
Secretary + Treasurer:	H.K.A. Visser (NL)
Council:	A. Prader (CH), J. Bierich (D), H. Andersen (DK), W. Hamilton (UK), R. François (F)
Participants (n):	21 members, 39 guests, 27 accompanying persons – Reg. Fee: USD 10
Abstracts (n):	36, published in Acta Paediatr Scand 1968;57:72–86

Scientific programme:
Perinatal endocrinology (C.A. and D.B. Villee: Placenta and foetal adrenal steroid synthesis); thyroid; steroids; adipose tissue and obesity (E. Shafrir: Hormonal aspects of adipose tissue metabolism); pituitary.

Social programme:
Annual Dinner at Hotel Shulamit, with Israeli folklore programme; Symposium: 'Child rearing in the Kibbutz'; Tour of Galilee (Nazareth, Tiberias, Kibbutz Ginosar, Capernaum, Akko); Tour Caesarea-Jerusalem (Hadassah University Hospital (Chagall windows), Yad Vashem, old city, Mt. Scopus, Dinner at King's Hotel/Mt. Zion, Israel Museum), Tel Aviv, Jaffa, Petah Tikva (Meet Israeli colleagues at home); Optional tour to the South of the country. – Ladies: Sightseeing Tour Haifa; Excursion to Megiddo.

Sponsors: Bank Haoalim, Chemie-Export Kontor, Choay, Ciba, Ikapharm, Kupat Holim, Merck, Sharp & Dohme, Nutritia, Organon, Sam-On, Schering.

1968 Vienna	7th Annual Meeting, Combined Meeting of ESPE and the European Club for Paediatric Research (= ESPR after 1969)
Date:	26th to 30th August
Venue:	Neues Institutsgebäude der Universität Wien, Vienna, Austria
President:	Walter Swoboda (A)
Secretary + Treasurer:	H.K.A. Visser (NL)
Council:	A. Prader (CH), J. Bierich (D), H. Andersen (DK), W. Hamilton (UK), R. François (F)
Participants (n):	159 (82 members, 77 guests, 44 accompanying persons) in total – ESPE: 66 (34 members, 32 guests), 27 accompanying persons – Reg. Fee: ATS 400
Abstracts (n):	59 (51 presented, 8 read by title), published in Acta Paediatr Scand 1969;58:191–207; – Meeting report (Z. Laron) Israel J Med Sci 1969;5:131

Scientific programme:
Calcium – Parathyroid – Thyrocalcitonine; Pancreas – Pituitary – Thyroid; Gonads – Adrenals.

Social programme:
Get-together visit to Belvedere Castle and Österreichische Galerie; Reception by the Lord Mayor of Vienna, visit to Schloss Schönbrunn; Congress Dinner at 'Le Palais',

introduced by the Vienna Philharmonia Schrammel Quartett; Heurigen visit in Grinzing. – Ladies: Sightseeing-tour through Vienna; Guided group visits to Hofburg, Treasure Chamber, National Library, Staatsoper, Petit Point Manufactury. Excursion to the Vienna Woods.

Sponsors:	Bayer Pharma, Ciba, Hoffmann-La Roche, Laevosan, Pfizer, Sandoz, Vedepha, Biochemie, Geigy, Kwizda, Organon, Richardson-Merrill, Schering, Dr. A. Wander, Werfft-Chemie.

1969 Malmö	**8th Annual Meeting, ESPE**
Date:	25th to 28th June
Venue:	Lecture Room, Department of Pathology, Malmö General Hospital, Malmö, Sweden
President:	Carl-Gustaf Bergstrand (S)
Secretary + Treasurer:	H.K.A. Visser (NL)
Council:	A. Prader (CH), Walter Teller (D), W. Hamilton (UK), R. François (F)
Participants (n):	71 (33 members, 3 corresponding members, 35 guests), 22 accompanying persons – Reg. Fee: USD 10
Abstracts (n):	38, published in Acta Paediatr Scand 1969;58:654-673

Scientific programme:
The child of the diabetic mother; Growth hormone and growth problems; Sex differentiation and sex anomalies (e.g. A. Jost: Hormonal factors in sex differentiation of the mammalian foetus); Steroids.

Social programme:
Reception by the City of Malmö at Town Hall; Evening tour to Lund (University, Cathedral with church music, supper at Stäket vaults); Annual Dinner at Hotel Kung Carl; Full day excursion to Skåne, visit to Ystad. – Ladies: Sightseeing in Skåne (castle visit, Kosta crystal); Tour of Malmö (Doll-House Shop, modern Swedish Day Nursery, fortress Malmöhus (ethnological exhibition), lunch at Kockska krogen.

Sponsors:	AB Semper, AB Findus, Ciba Produkter AB, AB Draco, Ferring AB, AB Ferrosan, San-bolagen AB, Svenska Hoechst AB, Upjohn AB.

1970 Lyon	**9th Annual Meeting, ESPE**
Date:	16th to 20th July
Venue:	South Amphitheatre, University of Medicine; Pasteur Institute; Lyon, France
President:	René François (F)
Secretary + Treasurer:	H.K.A. Visser (NL)
Council:	A. Prader (CH), W. Teller (D), W. Hamilton (UK), C.G. Bergstrand (S)
Participants (n):	98 (41 members, 2 corresponding members, 55 guests), 21 accompanying persons – Reg. Fee: USD 10
Abstracts (n):	46, published in Acta Paediatr Scand 1971;60:603–619

Scientific programme:
Fetal and neonatal endocrinology (e.g., E. Diczfalusy: Synthesis of steroids in human feto-placental unit, R.M. Blizzard: Maturation of fetal and neonatal thyroid function); Growth hormone; Thyroid; Endocrinology of puberty; Adrenal cortex; Round Tables: Androgen determination, Competitive binding techniques.

Social programme:
Get-together at the Museum of Medical History, then visit to the old part of Lyon; Reception by the Mayor at Hôtel de Ville, Dinner at Casino de Charbonnières; Annual Dinner in the Hôtel Dieu; Full day excursion to the Beaujolais region. – Ladies: Visit to old city of Perouges; Visit to the 'Rosarie', the museum of fabrics, the Roman theatre of Fourvière, the Cathedral of Ainay; Visit of the old city of Vienne, Rhone valley.

Sponsors:	Ciba, France-Lait, Insitut Merieux, Nativelle, Promedica, Solac, Sopad-Nestlé, UPSA

1971 Zurich	**10th Annual Meeting, ESPE**
Date:	8th to 12th May
Venue:	Kinderspital (Children's Hospital), University of Zurich, Switzerland
President:	José M. Francés (E)/Andrea Prader (CH)
Secretary + Treasurer:	H.K.A. Visser (NL)
Council:	W. Hamilton (UK), C.G. Bergstrand (S), W. Teller (D), Jean Bertrand (F), Pierre Ferrier (CH)
Participants (n):	138 (52 members, 3 corresponding members, 83 guests) – Reg. Fee: USD 20
Abstracts (n):	53 (10 read by title), published in Acta Paediatr Scand 1972; 61:243–270

Scientific programme:

Testosterone and testes (D. Knorr: Synthesis and metabolism of testosterone); Male pseudohermaphroditism; Congenital adrenal hyperplasia (A.M. Bongiovanni: Another look at CAH due to 3β-HSD deficiency); Normal and precocious puberty (R. Rappaport: Gonadal and adrenal activity at the initial stages of puberty); Hypothalamus-pituitary-thyroxid axis; Protein hormones; Free papers; Psycho-endocrinology (J. Money: Development of sexual identification, E.H. Wallis: Psychological management of children with intersexuality).

Social programme:

Get together; Excursion to Winterthur (Art collection Oskar Reinhart), to the Rheinfall, supper at Schloss Laufen; Reception by the City and Canton of Zurich at Muraltengut; Visit of Fraumünster cathedral (Chagall windows, organ recital), Annual Dinner at Guildhouse 'Zur Meise'; Full day excursion to the Rigi. – Accompanying persons: Visit of Einsiedeln church and monastery, lunch; Fashion lunch at Mövenpick Dreikönigshaus.

| Sponsors: | Ciba-Geigy, Dr. Bender & Dr. Hobein, Dr. A. Wander, Fluka, Hoechst-Pharma, F. Hoffmann-La Roche & Co, R. Hunter, Laboratorien Hausmann, Merck, Sharp & Dohme, Mettler Instrumente, Milian Instruments, Nestlé, Organon, Sandoz, Schering-Zürich; Schweiz. Serum- & Impfinstitut, Siegfried. |

1972 Louvain	**11th Annual Meeting, ESPE**
Date:	7th to 10th September
Venue:	Collège du Pape, Louvain, Belgium
President:	Paul Malvaux (B)
Secretary:	Milo Zachmann (CH)
Treasurer:	J. Leo Van den Brande (NL)
Council:	C.G. Bergstrand (S), W. Teller, J. Bertrand (F), P. Ferrier (CH)
Participants (n):	130 – Reg. Fee: BEF 1,000
Abstracts (n):	62 (9 read by title), published in Acta Paediatr Scand 1973;62:83–112

Scientific programme:

Steroids in infancy and childhood (C. Migeon: Transplacental passage of glucocorticoids in pregnancy near term); Congenital adrenal hyperplasia and other steroid disorders; Clinical investigations; Gonadotropin secretion and mechanism of puberty (J. Bertrand: Plasma oestrogens before puberty in human); Thyroid evaluation (D.E. Fisher: Thyroid function in the fetus and newborn); Somatomedin and growth

hormone; *Diabetes and hypoglycemia, *Long term effect of disease and of therapy, *Calcium metabolism and related problems; Free communications (G. Hers: Recent developments in the biochemistry of hormone action).
* Parallel session

Social programme:

Get-together (bar of the Collège du pape); Reception by the Rector of the Catholic University of Louvain, visit of the Grand Beguinage, Annual Dinner at the Faculty Club, Grand Beguinage; Reception at the Brussels City Hall at the Grand Place; Full day excursion to Brugge. – Ladies: Excursion to Brussels; Visit of Louvain and excursion to Brabant Wallon.

| Sponsors: | Nestlé-Guigoz, Nutricia, Organon Belge, Wellcome, Delagrange, Janssen Pharmaceutica, RIT, UCB, Abbott, Beecham, Bristol Benelux, Christiaens, Glaxo Benelux, Mead Johnson Benelux, Roche, Specia, Rodolphe Coles, Lepetit Belgica, Novo Industries, Sandoz. |

1973 Bergen	**12th Annual Meeting, ESPE**
Date:	21st to 24th June
Venue:	Studentsenteret (The Students' Centre), Bergen, Norway
President:	Dagfinn Aarskog (N)
Secretary:	M. Zachmann (CH)
Treasurer:	J.L. Van den Brande (NL)
Council:	J. Bertrand (F), P. Ferrier (CH), Dietrich Knorr (D)
Participants (n):	137 active (54 members, 3 corresponding members, 80 guests), 47 accompanying persons – Reg. Fee: NOK 250
Abstracts (n):	71 (23 read by title), published in Acta Paediatr Scand 1974;63:320–333

Scientific programme:

Long term effect of congenital adrenal hyperplasia (A. Bongiovanni: Adrenogenital syndrome: later consequences, J. Money: Behavioural outcome after early cortisone therapy in the adrenogenital syndrome of 46,XX hermaphroditism); Adrenocortical function; Normal and precocious puberty; Growth and growth hormone; Hypothalamo–pituitary–gonadal axis; Somatomedin; *Testosterone and Testes, *Free papers; *Glucagon – insulin – growth hormone, *Pituitary and pituitary function.
* 2 parallel sessions

Social programme:
Get-together at Sjøfartsmuseet (Maritime Museum); Reception by the City of Bergen and Annual Dinner at Håkonshallen; Midsummernight at Solstrand Fjord Hotel; Full day excursion: roundtrip 'Norway in a nutshell' – Accompanying persons: Visit of Troldhaugen, home of Edvard Grieg, with piano music, Fantoft Stavechurch, Funicular to Mt. Fløyen and lunch; Visit of the Leprosy museum and Bryggen centre for arts and crafts.

Sponsors: Astra-Gruppen, Barfods Pharmaceutiske A/S, Collett, Dumex, Eli Lilly, Ferring, Hoffmann-La Roche & Co., Kabi, Nestlé, Novo Industri, Organon, Pfizer, Sandoz, Schering Berlin, Schering Corp. USA.

1974 Paris	13th Annual Meeting, ESPE
Date:	12th to 15th September
Venue:	Amphitheatre, Hôpital des Enfants-Malades, Paris, France
President:	Pierre Royer (F)
Secretary:	M. Zachmann (CH)
Treasurer:	J.L. Van den Brande (NL)
Council:	D. Aarskog (N), J. Bertrand (F), D. Knorr (D), P. Malvaux (B)
Participants (n):	Around 200 – Reg. Fee: FRF 250
Abstracts (n):	65 (20 read by title), published in Pediatr Res 1975;9:680–690

Scientific programme:
Hormone receptors and growth hormone (J. Roth: GH receptors: new tools for studies in man); Adrenals; Neuroendocrinology (M.M. Grumbach and S.L. Kaplan: Advances in neuroendocrinology, clinical significance); Foetal endocrinology (A. Jost et al: Hormonal control of carbohydrate metabolism in foetal and neonatal liver); Somatomedin and cartilage (J.J. Van Wyk: The insulin-like and growth-promoting actions of somatomedin as revealed by membrane binding techniques); *Steroids, *Free papers; *Growth, *Hypothalamic-pituitary regulation; Testicular function and masculinisation (N. Josso: The anti-Müllerian hormone of the fetal testis).
* 2 parallel sessions

Social programme:
Get-together at Cloître de Port-Royal; Reception by the President of University René Descartes at the University Hall, then dance at Moulin de la Galette (Montmartre); Annual Dinner at Palais du Luxembourg; Excursion: Guided tour of the old Quartier du Marais, Lunch at local members' homes. – Ladies: Tour to the Castle of Vaux-le-Vicomte and Fontainebleau.

Sponsors: Ciba-Geigy, Jouillé, Nestlé, Organon, Roussel, Sandoz, Servier, Specia, Unilabo, Wellcome, Fondation de France, Fondation Mérieux, Syndicat National des Industries Pharmaceutiques, Assistance Publique de Paris, Ministère de la Santé, Ministère des Affaires Etrangères: Departement des Relations Culturelles, Université René Descartes Paris.

1975 Berlin	14th Annual Meeting, ESPE
Date:	24th to 27th September
Venue:	Klinikum Steglitz, Free University, Berlin, West Germany
President:	Hans Helge (D)
Secretary:	M. Zachmann (CH)
Treasurer:	J.L. Van den Brande (NL)
Council:	D. Aarskog (N), J. Bertrand (F), D. Knorr (D), P. Malvaux (B)
Participants (n):	Around 200 – Reg. Fee: DEM 160 (active), DEM 120 (accompanying)
Abstracts (n):	76 (28 read by title), published in Pediatr Res 1975;9:666–677

Scientific programme:
Juvenile diabetes mellitus (A. Drash: Modern concepts of juvenile diabetes mellitus, E.F. Pfeiffer: Artificial pancreas, J. Köbberling: Genetic heterogeneity within idiopathic diabetes, *A.P. Hansen: The effects of growth hormone and somatostatin in juvenile diabetics, A.S. Luyckx: The role of glucagon in juvenile-type diabetics, Z. Laron: Various faces of diabetes mellitus in childhood), *Steroids; *Diabetes mellitus, *Puberty; Drugs and hormone metabolism (A. Kappas: The heme system in relation to drug and hormone detoxification, W. Hamilton: The action of drugs on hormone biosynthesis and metabolism, B.L. Mirkin: The influence of drug therapy on steroid metabolism in childhood, M.I. New: Drug and hormone influence in childhood hypertension); *Growth hormone and growth, *Free papers; Neuroendocrine control (R. Bock: Functional morphology of the hypothalamus, W. Wuttke: Neuro-transmitters and hormone release, F. Ellendorff: Amygdala-hypothalamic transmission after neonatal hormone exposure, M. Schmidt-Gollwitzer: LH-RH secretion and gonadal function); *Hypothalamo-pituitary function, *Neonatal Endocrinology.
* 4 parallel sessions

Social programme:
Get-together (Brücke-Museum); Reception by the Senator of Health, Schloss Charlottenburg, Philharmonic Concert (R. Strauss conducted by Karajan) at Neue

Philharmonie (optional); Annual Dinner, Hotel Schweizerhof (Medieval Feast by Candlelight); Excursion: Berlin River Tour (Havel-Wannsee-Rundfahrt) followed by private invitations. – Ladies: Sightseeing Tour Berlin-West; Visit of 'Royal Prussian' Porcelain Manufacture (KPM).

Sponsors:	Senat von Berlin, Freie Universität Berlin, Medizinisch-Pharmazeutische Studiengesellschaft, Alldiät, Ciba-Geigy, Henning Berlin, Farbwerke Hoechst, Humana Milchwerke, Deutsche Kabi, Milupa, Merck, Novo Industrie, Schering, Serono.

1976 Rotterdam	15th Annual Meeting, ESPE – Joint Meeting with the European Society for Paediatric Research (ESPR) and the Working Group for Mineral Metabolism (WGMM)
Date:	20th to 24th June
Venue:	New Buildings, Medical Faculty, Erasmus University, Rotterdam, The Netherlands
President:	Hendrick K.A. Visser (NL)
Secretary:	M. Zachmann (CH)
Treasurer:	J.L. Van den Brande (NL)
Council:	J. Bertrand (F), P. Malvaux (B), Bruno Weber (D), Jaakko Perheentupa (FIN)
Participants (n):	Over 500 – Reg. Fee: NLG 185 (active), NLG 135 (accompanying)
Abstracts (n):	187 (oral and poster presentations), published in Pediatr Res 1976;10:874–904

Scientific programme:

R. Rappaport: Hormonal control of skeletal growth and metabolism, J.W. Hekkelman: Parathyroid hormone receptors and membrane functions; *Vitamin D, parathormone and bone metabolism (S. Balsan: Results of treatment with hydroxylated vitamin D derivatives in bone diseases), *Newborn pathophysiology (A. Huch: Transcutaneous measurement of arterial pO_2 in the newborn), *Hormones and growth: somatomedin and other growth factors; P (D.R. Fraser: Pathophysiology and treatment of the rachitic syndromes); *Secretion and action of parathormone (O.L.M. Bijvoet: Parathormone extracellular ion homeostasis and the kidney), *Newborn: bilirubin and photo therapy (A.L. Stewart: Follow-up of infants at high risk of mental and physical handicap), *Hormones and growth: growth hormone.

M. Winick: Nutritional problems in affluent societies: pediatric problems; *Nutrition of fetus and newborn (J. Metcoff: Intrauterine nutrition, cell function and growth),

*Endocrinology: adrenocortical steroids (M.I. New: Low renin hypertension and hypokalemia in a 3-years old girl with deficiency of all known steroids), *Hormones and growth: puberty; K. Hall: Somatomedins and some other growth factors, I.Pastan: The role of cyclic AMP in the control of growth and behaviour of cultured fibroblast cells; *W.B. Kannel: Atherosclerosis and pediatrics, *Fetal and neonatal endocrinology (G.D. Thorburn: Development of the fetal pituitary-adrenal system in animals), *Gastroenterology and intestinal enzymes; (R.D.G. Milner: Fetal and neonatal endocrinology: clinical aspects; *Various subjects, *Growth: clinical subjects, *Metabolism: carbohydrates.

D. De Wied: Pituitary hormones and motivational, learning and memory processes; *Releasing hormones (M. Besser: GH release inhibiting hormone, somatostatin), *Genetics and metabolism (D. Bootsma: Somatic cell genetics and congenital disease), *Developmental pharmacology; (P.E. Polani: Role of the sex chromosomes in the determination of sex in mammals, C. Hutt: Biological basis of psychological sex differences); *Sexual differentiation, *Metabolism: amino acids, *Developmental biology.
* Parallel sessions

Social programme:
Get-together (Museum Boymans Van Beuningen); Concert at Laurens Church by 'Concerto Rotterdam'; Half day excursion to Amsterdam; Farewell dinner party at 'De Doelen'. – Accompanying persons: Rotterdam sightseeing tour; Excursion to miniature town Madurodam; Show of ancient Dutch fashions 1540–1940.

| Sponsors: | Astra, Ciba-Geigy, Hoechst, Kabi, Merck, Milupa, Nestlé, Nordisk Insulinlaboratorium, Novo Industrie, Organon, Sandoz, Serono, Schering Berlin, Wellcome. |

1977 Cambridge	16th Annual Meeting, ESPE
Date:	14th to 17th September
Venue:	King's College and Mill Lane Lecture Theatres, University of Cambridge, UK
President:	Charles G.D. Brook (UK)
Secretary:	M. Zachmann (CH)
Treasurer:	J.L. Van den Brande (NL)
Council:	David Grant (UK), J. Perheentupa (FIN), Raphaël Rappaport (F), B. Weber (D)
Participants (n):	195 active, 55 accompanying persons – Reg. Fee: GBP 90 active, GBP 80 accompanying persons (including, e.g. punting on the river Cam)
Abstracts (n):	87 (44 oral presentations, 29 posters, 14 read by title), published in Pediatr Res 1978;12:148–166

Scientific programme:

Gastrointestinal hormones (S.R. Bloom); Foetal and neonatal endocrinology; Growth and growth hormone; Male intersex conditions (A. Prader); Control of FSH secretion in men and boys (H.S. Jacobs); Growth factors; Thyroid screening and disorders; Intracellular events underlying insulin secretion (L. Orci); Clinical session.

Social programme:

Reception in King's College, organ recital in King's College Chapel; Conference Banquet in King's College, followed by Concert in King's College Chapel: The English Chamber Orchestra featuring Murray Peraia as soloist; Excursion: Audley End House at Saffron Walden, Lavenham, Bury St. Edwards.

| Sponsors: | Marks & Spencer Ltd., Glaxo Holdings Ltd., Ames Co., Pharmacia G.B., Panax Equipment Ltd. |

1978 Athens	17th Annual Meeting, ESPE
Date:	10th to 13th September
Venue:	Apollon Palace Hotel, Kavouri (25 km off Athens centre), Greece
President:	Catherine Dacou-Voutetakis (GR)
Secretary:	R. Rappaport (F)
Treasurer:	P.C. Sizonenko (CH)
Council:	D. Grant (UK), J. Perheentupa (FIN), B. Weber (D)
Participants (n):	109 active – Reg. Fee: USD 80 active, USD 60 accompanying persons
Abstracts (n):	114 (45 oral presentations, 29 posters, 40 read by title), published in Pediatr Res 1978;12:1083–1104

Scientific programme:

Pineal hormones (R.J. Wurtman); Steroid receptors in the brain (M. Warembourg); Impact of immunology in endocrinology (A.M. DiGeorge); HLA linkage of 21-OH-deficiency; Oral insulin (G. Gregoriadis).

Social programme:

'Get-together-cruise' in the Saronian Gulf to islands of Aegina, Poros and Hydra; Concert: Thessaloniki State Orchestra (Herodes Atticus Theatre) or folk dances (Dora Stratou Theatre); Annual Dinner; Full day bus excursion: Mycenae, Epidaurus, Nafplia. – Accompanying Persons: Visit to Akropolis and walk through Plaka to Monasteraki; Excursion to Cape Sounion.

| Sponsors: | Nordisk Insulinlaboratorium, AB Kabi, Novo Daphni Co., Organon Hellas, Ni-The, Ferring Pharmaceuticals, Abbott, Wellcome. |

1979 Ulm	18th Annual Meeting, ESPE
Date:	20th to 23rd June
Venue:	Edwin-Scharff-Haus Congress Centre, Neu-Ulm, West Germany
President:	Walter W. Teller (D)
Secretary:	R. Rappaport (F)
Treasurer:	P.C. Sizonenko (CH)
Council:	Frank Bidlingmaier (D), C. Dacou-Voutetakis (GR), D. Grant (UK), Martin Ritzén (S)
Participants (n):	approx. 200 – Reg. Fee: DEM 70 active, DEM 50 accompanying persons
Abstracts (n):	85 (48 oral presentations, 20 poster, 17 read by title), published in Pediatr Res 1979;13:1184–1200.

Scientific programme:
Recent advances in perinatal thyroidology (D.A. Fisher); Calcium homeostasis, vitamin D metabolism and parathormone in childhood (R. Ziegler); Development and perinatal function of the adrenal cortex (C.H.L. Shackleton); Recent advances in the aetiology, pathophysiology and control of juvenile diabetes mellitus (K.D. Hepp).

Social programme:
Get together City museum; Organ concert in the cathedral (Ulmer Münster); Annual Dinner at Kornhaus; Full day bus excursion: Upper Suebia and Lake Konstanz. – Ladies: Sightseeing walk city of Ulm; visit bread museum; Bus tour: medieval architecture in South Germany.

Sponsors:	Carl Abt KG, Nestlé-Alpenmilch, Bayer AG, Befelka, H. Bessler, Ciba-Geigy, Daimler-Benz, Deutsche Kabi, Drägerwerk, Galenika Hetterich, Hoechst AG, Hormon Chemie, Humana Milchwerke, Maizena, E. Merck AG, L. Merckle KG, Milupa AG, Organon, Paul-Martini-Stiftung, A. Roussel Pharma, Sandoz, Serono, Schering AG.

1980 Bergamo	19th Annual Meeting, ESPE
Date:	31st August to 3rd September
Venue:	Seminario Papa Giovanni XXIII Congress Centre, Bergamo, Italy
President:	Giuseppe Chiumello (I)
Secretary:	R. Rappaport (F)
Treasurer:	P.C. Sizonenko (CH)
Council:	F. Bidlingmaier (D), C. Dacou-Voutetakis (GR), D. Grant (UK), M. Ritzén (S)

| Participants (n): | 200–250 – Reg. Fee: ITL 68,000 active, ITL 53,000 accompanying persons |
| Abstracts (n): | 101 (50 oral presentations, 36 poster, 15 read by title), published in Pediatr Res 1981;15:74–94 |

Scientific programme:
Recombinant DNA and endocrinology (J.D. Baxter); Postpubertal amenorrhea (P.G. Crosignani); Update of CAH (M.I. New); Developmental aspects of insulin and glucagon receptors (M.A. Sperling).

Social programme:
Get-together at Palazzo della Regione (Upper Town); Organ concert at Basilica di Santa Maria Maggiore; Annual Dinner at Castello di Malpaga; Excursion to Lake Como (bus and boat), visit of Villa Carlotta and Bellagio, lunch in Menaggio. – Ladies: Sightseeing walk of Upper Town, bus trip into countryside; Visit of 'Accademia Carrara' art gallery.

| Sponsors: | Various Italian banks, Hoechst Italia, Humana Italia, Mellin, Miles Italia, Nestlé, Plasmon-Dieterba, Serono Symposia. |

1981 Geneva	**20th Meeting, ESPE – 1st Joint Meeting with the Lawson Wilkins Pediatric Endocrine Society (LWPES)**
Date:	9th to 11th September
Venue:	New Building, Uni II, Université de Genève, Geneva, Switzerland
President:	Pierre C. Sizonenko (CH)
Secretary:	R. Rappaport (F)
Treasurer:	P.C. Sizonenko (CH)
Council:	F. Bidlingmaier (D), G. Chiumello (I), D. Grant (UK), M. Ritzén (S)
Participants (n):	241 active, 62 accompanying persons – Reg. Fee: CHF 200 active, CHF 150 accompanying persons
Abstracts (n):	207 (64 oral presentations, 116 poster, 27 read by title), published in Pediatr Res 1981;15:1538–1575

Scientific programme:
Screening of congenital hypothyroidism; Lipotrophins, endorphins and enkephalins (L. Rees); Neuroendocrinology; IGFs in vitro and in vivo (J. Zapf); Growth, growth hormone and somatomedins (L.E. Underwood); Somatomedins throughout development (V. Sara); Hormonal control of cartilage metabolism (M.T. Corvol); New

aspects of carbohydrate and lipid metabolism: Metabolic fuel transport (D.M. Bier), Metabolism in carbohydrate disorders (J.M. Olefsky), Fuel homeostasis and insulin resistance (A. DeFronzo), Endocrine and metabolic changes due to hypothalamic manipulations (B. Jeanrenaud); *Lawson-Wilkins-Lecture*: Calcium and cAMP as synarchic messengers (H. Rasmussen); Neural crest histogenesis of endocrine glands (N. LeDouarin); Physiology and pathology of peptide hormone receptors (K.J. Catt).

Social programme:
Get-together reception, Concert by the Quatuor of Geneva, Annual Dinner at Noga Hilton Hotel, Excursion: Lake Geneva boat trip, Nyon castle and Roman museum. – Accompanying persons: Guided tour of Old Town, Excursion to Abbey of Romainmôtier (lunch, organ concert), Visit to International Red Cross Committee or to Library Bodmeriania Bibliotheca.

Sponsors: University and School of Medicine of Geneva, Swiss Academy of Medical Sciences, Swiss National Science Foundation, Geneva Academic Society; AG Leo, Eli Lilly, Genentech, Hausmann Labs, Hoechst AG, Interpharma, Nestlé Nutrition, Opopharma SA, Organon, Schering AG, Smith Kline & French, Syntex Pharma, Zyma SA.

1982 Helsinki	21st Annual Meeting, ESPE
Date:	28th June to 1st July
Venue:	Great Hall, University, and Porthania Congress Centre, Helsinki, Finland
President:	Jaakko Perheentupa (FIN)
Secretary:	R. Rappaport (F)
Treasurer:	P.C. Sizonenko (CH)
Council:	Albert Aynsley-Green (UK), G. Chiumello (I), Wolfgang G. Sippell (D), Magda Vanderschueren-Lodeweyckx (B)
Participants (n):	approx. 220 – Reg. Fee: FIM 520 per person
Abstracts (n):	129 (44 oral, 50 poster presentations, 35 read by title), published in Pediatr Res 1982;16:886–907

Scientific programme:
Screening for congenital hypothyroidism; Symposium 1: Maturation and regulation of the testis (K. Purvis: Maturation of Leydig cell function, M. Ritzén: Regulation of Sertoli cell function, N.E. Skakkebaek: Carcinoma in situ of the testis – its relation to cryptorchidism, M.A. Rivarola: Intratesticular steroid hormone metabolism, M. Forest: Effects of hCG on the human testis and its application as a Leydig cell function test); *Testis, *Free papers; Symposium 2: Ethical problems (D. Aarskog: Ethics of

prenatal diagnosis in 21-hydroxylase deficiency and gonosome abnormalities, R. Rappaport: Ethical aspects of modifying normal growth, K. Kouvalainen: Ethics in paediatric research in relation to the Helsinki declaration); *Puberty, *Water and salt metabolism; Immunological aspects in paediatric endocrinology (G.F. Bottazzo); *Thyroid, *Immunology; *Growth factors 1, *Steroids; Neuroendocrine factors in the pathophysiology of obesity (J.M. Martin); *Growth factors 2, *Diabetes.
* Parallel sessions

Social programme:
Reception in City Hall; Concert in Church-in-the-Rock; Annual dinner at Forest Lake Hotel, preceded by open-air artistic programme or sauna and swimming in the lake; Excursion: Boat trip through archipelago to Haikko Manor, after lunch bus to medieval town of Porvoo. – Accompanying persons: Finnish traditions: handicrafts, open air museum; Sibelius tour to Ainola and to studio of painter Halonen.

Sponsors:	The Jusélius Foundation, Chymos, Ferring AB, Hoechst AG, KabiVitrum AB, Leiras Pharmaceuticals, Miles Labs, Nordisk Insulinlaboratorium, Novo Industri A/S, Orion Diagnostica, Remeda Pharmaceutical, The Upjohn Company.

1983 Budapest	22nd Annual Meeting, ESPE
Date:	30th August to 1st September
Venue:	Cultural Centre, Budapest, Hungary
President:	Ferenc Péter (H)
Secretary:	A. Aynsley-Green (UK)
Treasurer:	P.C. Sizonenko (CH)
Council:	Jean-Louis Chaussain (F), G. Chiumello (I), W.G. Sippell (D), M. Vanderschueren-Lodeweyckx (B)
Participants (n):	approx. 200 – Reg. Fee: USD 150 active, USD 100 accompanying persons
Abstracts (n):	113 (45 oral, 33 poster presentations, 35 read by title), published in Pediatr Res 1984;18:101–120

Scientific programme:
Thyroid (A. Burger: Alterations of thyroid hormone metabolism in disease, B. Rees-Smith: Immunoendocrinological aspects of the TSH receptor); *Adrenal, *Growth hormone and growth factors 1; Gastrointestinal hormones (A. Aynsley-Green: The role of hormones in the adaptation of the human newborn infant to postnatal nutrition); *Gonads, *Carbohydrate metabolism; LHRH and analogues (K. Nikolics: Biochemistry of LHRH and analogues, J. Happ: Treatment with GnRH and its potent analogs); * Thyroid, *GH and growth factors 2; Hypothalamic hormones (D. Fisher:

Neurohypophyseal peptides in the perinatal period); Corpus pineale (B. Mess: Endocrine role of the pineal gland in the reproduction of experimental animals, D. Gupta: Melatonin in children, U. Lang: Melatonin retards sexual maturation).
* Parallel sessions

Social programme:
Get-together party at Hotel Forum; Folk music and dances, Annual Banquet at Restaurant Gundel; Concert at Budavari Lutheran Church; Full day excursion to Esztergom and Szentendre at the Danube Bend.

Sponsors: Chemical Works Gedeon Richter Ltd., Ferring GmbH, Hoechst AG, Kabivitrum AB, Serono.

1984 Heidelberg	23rd Annual Meeting, ESPE
Date:	2nd to 5th September
Venue:	Theoretikum, University of Heidelberg, West Germany
President:	Dieter Schönberg (D)
Secretary:	A. Aynsley-Green (UK)
Treasurer:	Michel L. Aubert (CH)
Council:	J.L. Chaussain (F), Agne Larsson (S), W.G. Sippell (D), M. Vanderschueren-Lodeweyckx (B)
Participants (n):	approx. 300 – Reg. Fee: DEM 300 active, DEM 200 accompanying persons
Abstracts (n):	146 (52 oral, 94 poster presentations in 15 guided tours), published in Pediatr Res 1984;18:1206–1232

Scientific programme:
Non-radioactive methods for the determination of hormones; Molecular biochemistry (G. Schütz: Receptor function at cellmembrane, signal conversion to second messenger, F. Hofmann: Second messenger to effect on intracellular receptor); *Brain and puberty, *CAH and adrenal hormones; Hypophysiotropic neuropeptides (J. Spiess); *Growth hormones, *Puberty; Diabetes mellitus (J. Nerup: Concepts of pathophysiology in diabetes, A. Drash: Clinical aspects and epidemiology of diabetes); *Somatomedins, *Diabetes mellitus, hGH; Clinical use of releasing hormones (F. Labrie); *Steroid hormones, *Diagnostic procedures.
* Parallel sessions

Social programme:
Reception at Heidelberg Town-Hall, Tour through Kurpfälzisches Museum; Concert (Southwest German Chamber Orchestra) at Old University Aula; Annual Dinner at

Heidelberg Castle; Full day boat tour on the Neckar to Eberbach, visit of Guttenberg Castle. – Accompanying persons: Tours to Roman Town Ladenburg, to the Barock Castle of Schwetzingen, to old Celtic Heiligenberg, to medieval Monastery of Maulbronn, to Barock Residency of Bruchsal or to Bauhaus Centre of Art Deco at Darmstadt.

Sponsors: Amersham-Buchler, Behring-Werke, Laboratorien Berthold, Bio-Rad Laboratories, Boehringer Mannheim, Henning Berlin, Hoechst AG, Humana Milchwerke, Joyce Loebl Düsseldorf, Deutsche Kabi-Vitrum, Eli Lilly, Milupa AG, Nordisk-Deutschland, E. Merck Darmstadt, Organon, Sandoz AG Nürnberg.

1985 Baltimore	24th Annual Meeting, ESPE – 2nd Joint Meeting with the LWPES
Date:	22nd to 26th June
Venue:	Hyatt Regency Hotel, Baltimore, Maryland, USA
President:	Raphaël Rappaport (F)
Secretary:	A. Aynsley-Green (UK)
Treasurer:	M.L. Aubert (CH)
Council:	J.L. Chaussain (F), A. Larsson (S), Michael B. Ranke (D), Jean-Pierre Bourguignon (B)
Participants (n):	not available – Reg. Fee: USD 180 members, USD 210 non-members, USD 30 fellows (scientific program only), USD 130 spouses
Abstracts (n):	200 (40 oral, 160 poster presentations), published in Pediatr Res 1985;19:603–637

Scientific programme:
W. Vale: Hypophysiotropic regulatory peptides; *GRF, diabetes insipidus and thyroid; *Puberty, sexual differentation; GRF (P. Brazeau: Somatostatin and somatocrinin, L. Frohman: Physiologic and pharmacokinetic studies with GRF, R. Blizzard: Therapeutic effects of GRF); *Lawson-Wilkins-Lecture:* Insulin-like growth factors: an update (R.E. Humbel); *Adrenal, carbohydrate metabolism; *Growth factors; Adrenal (J. Laragh: The renin axis and the natriuretic hormone in electrolyte and blood pressure homeostasis: pathophysiologic implications, R. Carey: Aldosterone stimulating factor: a newly recognized hormone, I. Reid: Actions of angiotensin II on the brain).

G.F. Bottazzo: Endocrine autoimmunity: a review; Diabetes (N.K. Maclaren: Inherited susceptibility to insulin dependent diabetes mellitus, G.S. Eisenbarth: Type I diabetes: chronic progressive autoimmune disease: prediction of onset and immunotherapy trials, P.E. Lacy: Present status of islet transplant in diabetes); *Calcium – parathyroid

(M.T. Corvol: Chondrocyte differentiation and vitamin D, F. Glorieux: Hormonal modulation of bone remodelling, A.M. Spiegel: Pseudohypoparathyroidism: hormone resistance caused by defects in the receptor adenylate cyclase complex); *LRF (M. Henzl: Long term effects of LRF agonists on gonadal function, M.M. Grumbach: Pathophysiology and treatment of true precocious puberty, W.F. Crowley: Long term effects upon growth and development of LHRH analogue suppression of puberty, S.L.S. Drop, J.L. Chaussain: Clinical studies with LRF in precocious puberty).
* Concurrent sessions

Social programme:
Reception at Baltimore Museum of Art; Peabody Conservatory of Music: recital and reception; Boat trip to Annapolis (historic buildings, US Naval Academy); Annual Banquet with dining and dancing; Home entertainment for overseas guests. – Accompanying persons: Tour of Historic Baltimore.

Sponsors: Genentech, Serono, KabiVitrum, Nichols Institute, Ross Laboratories, Nordisk, Ames, Pfizer, Pharmacia, Hoechst, Sanofi, Sandoz, Clin Midy, Merieux, Ferring, Beaufour Laboratoire.

1986 Zurich	25th Annual Meeting, ESPE
Date:	31th August to 3rd September
Venue:	Kinderspital (Children's Hospital) and University of Zurich, Switzerland
President:	Ruth Illig (CH)
Secretary:	A. Aynsley-Green (UK)
Treasurer:	M.L. Aubert (CH)
Council:	Maguelone G. Forest (F), A. Larsson (S), M.B. Ranke (D), J.P. Bourguignon (B)
Participants (n):	410 active, 90 accompanying – Reg. Fee: CHF 300 active, CHF 200 accompanying persons
Abstracts (n):	213 (51 oral, 129 poster, 33 read by title), oral+poster published in Pediatr Res 1986;20:1178–1208

Scientific programme:
Round table on human growth hormone; A. Prader: Growth – auxiological and endocrine aspects; *Growth, tall stature, delayed puberty; *Fetal, pre/perinatal endocrinology. Feto-placental endocrinology (M.L. Casey: The initiation of parturition, P. Siiteri: Function of progesterone in pregnancy maintenance, G. Mulder: The role of decidual PRL in ion and water transport across the fetal membranes, P. Bischof: Pregnancy associated plasma protein A). *Human growth hormone; *Congenital adrenal hyperplasia. *Androgens, gonads, intersex; *Growth factors, peptides. J.M. Polak: Regulatory peptides in

health and disease. *Precocious puberty, LHRH agonist; *Diabetes mellitus. Calcium-phosphorus metabolism (K. Kruse: Laboratory assessment of bone and mineral metabolism in childhood, S. Balsan: New aspects of vitamin D metabolism – hereditary resistance to 1,25-hydroxyvitamin D and its treatment, J. Fischer: Pseudohypoparathyroidism – circulating inhibitor and defect of receptor cyclase protein).
* Parallel sessions

Social programme:
Get-together party at Kinderspital; Concert by Johannes Kobelt Quartett, then Reception by City and Canton at Casino Zürichhorn; Annual banquet and dance at University Terrace and Lichthof; Full day excursion: special train to Maienfeld in the Rhine Valley 'Bündner Herrschaft' with mountain walk followed by picnic in an alpine meadow. – Accompanying persons: citytours, visits of museums, shopping, visit of chocolate factory.

Sponsors: Kanton und Stadt Zürich, Schweiz. Akademie der Medizin. Wissenschaften, Schweiz. Gesellschaft für Endokrinologie, Schweiz. Ges. für Pädiatrie; Beckmann Instruments, Boehringer Mannheim, Buehlmann Laboratories, Eli Lilly, Ferring, Glaxo, Globopharm/KabiVitrum, Henning Berlin, Hoechst, Laboratorien Hausmann, Merck, Sharp & Dohme-Chibret, Nestlé Produkte, Nordisk, Packard Instruments, Rahn/Tschaeppeler, Sandoz, Sanofi, Schering, Schwabe Verlag, Schweiz. Bankverein, Swissair, Ares-Serono, Wild & Leitz.

1987 Toulouse	26th Annual Meeting, ESPE
Date:	6th to 8th September
Venue:	Faculté de Pharmacie, Université Paul Sabatier, Toulouse-Rangueil, France
President:	Pierre Rochiccioli (F)
Secretary:	A. Aynsley-Green (UK)
Treasurer:	M.L. Aubert (CH)
Council:	M.G. Forest (F), M.B. Ranke (D), Paul Czernichow (F), Ieuan A. Hughes (UK), President-elect: Niels E. Skakkebæk (DK)
Participants (n):	450 active, 150 accompanying persons – Reg. Fee: FRF 1200 active, FRF 800 accompanying persons
Abstracts (n):	232 (65 oral, 138 poster, 29 read by title), oral+poster published in Pediatr Res 1988;23:105–139

Scientific programme:
Non-conventional indications of hGH therapy (R. Rosenfeld: Turner's syndrome, G. Van Vliet: Constitutional short stature, W.G. Sippell: Partial GH deficiency); *Growth

hormone secretion, *Thyroid gland; H.A. Drexhage: Paediatric aspects of endocrine autoimmunity; *Growth Factors, Gonads – androgens; *Cushing´s syndrome, *Neonatal hyperinsulinism; *GHRH, *Water and salt metabolism; W. Wehrenberg: Regulation of GH secretion by GHRH and SRIH; *Precocious puberty – puberty, *Cranial irradiation – chondrocytes; E. Clauser: Human insulin receptor cDNA and its potential pathological expression; *hGH-therapy – Somatostatin, *Diabetes mellitus.
* Parallel sessions

Social programme:
Get-together Buffet; Concert by the Orchestre de Chambre de Toulouse, Reception at Musée des Augustins; Banquet at Hotel Dieu Saint Jacques; Full day excursion to Carcassonne and Cathar Chateaux. – Accompanying persons: Guided walk around the old city; Guided walk around the Renaissance Hotels.

Sponsors: Choay-Sanofi, KabiVitrum, Serono, Nordisk, Eli Lilly, Sarget, Ipsen, Ferring, Evian, Leo, Miles, Crinex, Hoechst, Bristol, Oris.

1988 Copenhagen	27th Annual Meeting, ESPE
Date:	26th to 29th June
Venue:	The Panum Institute, Copenhagen, Denmark
President:	Niels E. Skakkebæk (DK)
Secretary:	I.A. Hughes (UK)
Treasurer:	M. Aubert (CH)
Council:	Kerstin Albertsson-Wikland (S), P. Czernichow (F), M.G. Forest (F), Jan-Maarten Wit (NL), President-elect: Zvi Laron (IL)
Participants (n):	350 active – Reg. Fee: DKK 1,500 active, DKK 1,100 accompanying persons
Abstracts (n):	173 (50 oral, 123 poster presentations in 14 guided tours), published in Pediatr Res 1988;24:517–548

Scientific programme:
S. Ratcliffe: Growth and development of children with sex chromosome disorders; *Growth and development in Children Treated for Cancer (S. Shalet: ALL or brain tumours, D. Mosier: Growth in the head-irradiated rat, N. Barnes: Thyroid dysfunction following irradiation, J. Sanders: Bone marrow transplantation, M. Thorén: Stereotactic irradiation for pituitary disease, P. Clayton: Gonadal function, J. Müller: Gonadal morphology, P. Morris-Jones: Oncological trends and potential endocrine sequelae); *Diabetes, *Adrenals; *Thyroid; *Andrea-Prader-Lecture:* Milo Zachmann;

D. De Kretser: Inhibin, R. Sharpe: Regulation of testicular function, J. Rajfer: Treatment of cryptorchidism, *C.J.G. Wensing: Embryology of testicular descent, M.B. Jackson: Epidemiology of cryptorchidism, N.E. Skakkebæk: Neoplasia and cryptorchidism, H. Høstrup: Natural history of the maldescended testis, J.C. Job: Endocrine and immunological findings in the cryptorchid infant, S.M.P. de Muinck Keizer-Schrama: Hormonal treatment of cryptorchidism, P. Christiansen: Treatment of cryptorchidism: hCG or GnRH. A double-blind controlled study of 243 boys; A. Bergh: Acute 'inflammatory' effects of hCG on the rat testis, F. Hadziselimovic: GnRH effect on spermatogenesis in the cryptorchid testis. *Growth factors; *Growth hormone – biological aspects; *Growth hormone – secretion.
* Parallel sessions

Social programme:
Get-together party at Søpavillonen; Annual Banquet at Restaurant 'Nimb'; Annual excursion to North Zealand (Dyrehaven park, lunch at 'Bakken') – Accompanying persons: Royal tour of Copenhagen; visit to Royal Porcelain Factory.

Sponsors: Danish Cancer Society, Danish Medical Research Council, Ely Lilly, KabiVitrum, Nordisk Gentofte, Novo, Serono.

1989 Jerusalem	28th Annual Meeting, ESPE – 3rd Joint Meeting with the LWPES
Date:	29th October to 3rd November
Venue:	Hilton Hotel, Jerusalem, Israel
President:	Zvi Laron (IL)/S. Frazier (USA)
Secretary:	I.A. Hughes (UK)
Council:	K. Albertsson-Wikland (S), P. Czernichow (F), Peter Heidemann (D), J.-M. Wit (NL)
Participants (n):	942 – Reg. Fee: USD 260 active, USD 160 accompanying persons
Abstracts (n):	312 (94 oral, 218 poster presentations in 10 guided tours), published in Horm Res 1989;31(suppl 1):1–78

Scientific programme:
W.J. Rietveld: Chronobiology; *Lawson-Wilkins-Lecture:* Epidermal growth factor in developing mammals (D.A. Fisher); Immunological aspects of diabetes – update (G.S. Eisenbarth: Testing a 'linear' model for the prediction of type 1 diabetes, D. Elias: Anti-idiotypic networks in the pathogenesis and control of autoimmune diabetes, J. Dupré: Pathophysiology of cyclosporine-induced remission of IDDM); *Diabetes, glucose metabolism, *Puberty pathophysiology, *Growth hormone and IGF binding proteins.

Z. Naor: The GnRH receptor and signal transduction; Hormone action at the receptor and post-receptor level (E. Milgrom: The progesterone receptor, M. Kaufman: Androgen-receptor complexes, E. Karnieli: Glucose transporters in diabetes); Mode of action of GH and IGF (W.I. Wood: Purification, cloning and expression of the rabbit and human growth hormone receptors, O.G.P. Isaksson: Direct action of GH on cartilage, R.L. Hintz: The role of GH and IGF binding proteins, M.T. Corvol: IGF1 interaction with cartilage cells in vitro); *Growth – basic aspects, *Congenital adrenal hyperplasia, *Thyroid; Update on hGH – clinical aspects (M.A. Preece: Safety of GH treatment, J.L. Mills: Epidemiological aspects of undesirable effects of GH, K. Albertsson-Wikland: Definitions of GH insufficiency by physiological tests, E.O. Reiter: Definition of GH deficiency by pharmacological tests, C.G.D. Brook: Non-conventional use of growth hormone, R.G. Rosenfeld: Non-conventional GH therapy in Turner syndrome); *Andrea-Prader-Lecture:* Leo Van den Brande; *Laron-type dwarfism, GH-RH and hGH gene deletion, *Growth and sexual maturation, *Neuroendocrinology; *GH therapy, *Intersex – gonadal dysgenesis, *Pituitary tumours.

* Parallel sessions

Proceedings published in Horm Res 1990;33:45–160

Social programme:

Get-together reception; Opening ceremony with musical interlude and singer Shuli Natan; Oriental buffet reception and musical entertainment at Main Square, Jewish Quarter, Old City followed by sound & light show at David's Citadel; Banquet 'Wein, Weib, Gesang' at Jerusalem Convention Center; Full day excursion: Judean Desert, Wadi Kelt Monastery, lunch at Ein Gedi, dip in the Dead Sea, Massada mountain fortress, Bedouin-style buffet dinner at Ein Gedi. – Accompanying persons: Tour of Jerusalem and Yad Vashem; visit of Kibbutz Tsora and the Abshalom stalactite caves.

Sponsors:	Municipality of Jerusalem, Ares Serono, Eli Lilly International, Fujisawa Pharmaceutical Co., Kabi Peptide Hormones, Novo Nordisk A/S, Sanofi Recherche, Genentech Inc., Nichols Instiute, Serono Laboratories Inc., Hoechst AG, Levant X-Ray Ltd., Merck, Sharp & Dohme International; Teva Pharmaceutical Industries Ltd.
Organising Company:	Kenes Ltd., Tel Aviv, Israel

1990 Vienna	**29th Annual Meeting, ESPE**
Date:	2nd to 5th September
Venue:	Juridicum der Universität Wien, Vienna, Austria
President:	Herwig Frisch (A)
Secretary:	I.A. Hughes (UK)
Treasurer:	M.L. Aubert (CH)
Council:	K. Albertsson-Wikland (S), Michel Binoux (F), P. Heidemann (D), J.-M. Wit (NL); President-elect: V. Hesse (DDR)
Participants (n):	approx. 600 – Reg. Fee: ATS 2500 active, ATS 1600 accompanying persons
Abstracts (n):	244 (54 oral, 190 poster presentations in 11 guided tours), published in Horm Res 1990;33 (suppl 3):1–68

Scientific programme:

Methods of growth hormone estimation (P. Berger: Antigenic topography of GH, S. Woodhead: Quality controls for assays, J. Girard: How to interpret GH levels obtained with different assay systems, T. Torresani: GH estimation in urine, W. Blum: IGF and its binding proteins, Z. Hochberg: The GH binding protein, R. Rosenfeld: IGF- and GH-receptors); Endocrinology of puberty (S.R. Ojeda: Regulation of neuropeptide gene expression during puberty, T. Plant: The hypothalamic pulse generator, J.L. Cameron: Metabolic factors and sexual maturation, J.P. Bourguignon: Relevance of animal studies for the management of disorders of human puberty); *Puberty I, *IGF and binding proteins; *Puberty II, *GH deficiency: Therapy I, *Neuroendocrinology; J. Imperato-McGinley: Differentiation of gender identity; Endocrinology and immunology (H. Besedovsky: Interactions between the immune and the neuroendocrine systems, G. Wick: Disturbed immuno-endocrine feedback mechanisms in autoimmune disease, G.F. Bottazzo: Immunological basis of endocrine disorders); *GH physiology and secretion, *Androgens, intersex; *Immunology, *GH deficiency: Therapy II, *Adrenals; M.C. Sheppard: Genetic control of endocrine function; *Andrea-Prader-Lecture:* Raphael Rappaport.
* Parallel sessions

Social programme:

Get-together Reception by the Mayor of Vienna at Wappensaal, Wiener Rathaus; Concert given by members of the Vienna Philharmonic Orchestra at Palais Ferstel; Festive banquet (cocktail, gala dinner, dance) at Palais Schwarzenberg; Full day excursion to the Wachau valley (Benedictine monastery at Melk, lunch, by Danube steamer downstream to Dürnstein village and castle).

Sponsors:	Ares Serono, Eli Lilly, KabiVitrum, Novo Nordisk, Sanofi Pharma, Bissendorf Peptide, Erste Österreichische Spar Casse, Milupa Austria, Nestlé Austria, Sandoz, Wellcome.
Organising Company:	Vienna Medical Academy; Mondial Travel, Vienna

1991 Berlin	30th Annual Meeting, ESPE
Date:	25th to 28th August
Venue:	Congress Hall, Alexanderplatz, Berlin, Germany
President:	Volker Hesse (D)
Secretary:	I.A. Hughes (UK)
Treasurer:	M.L. Aubert (CH)
Council:	P. Czernichow (F), Stenvert L.S. Drop (NL), P. Heidemann (D), Niels E. Skakkebæk (DK); President-elect: A. Ferrández Longás (E)
Participants (n):	750 – Reg. Fee: DEM 350 active, DEM 250 accompanying persons
Abstracts (n):	220 (66 oral, 154 poster presentations in 21 guided tours), published in Horm Res 1991;35(suppl 2):1–62

Scientific programme:
Immunopathogenesis of type I diabetes (M.R. Christie: 64K antibodies, I. Ludwigsson: ICA and IAA in family studies, G.J. Bruining: ICA in population studies, I. Deschamps: Genetic polymorphism, E. Gale: Islet cell function, *Round Table:* Indication of future disease in healthy subjects); I. Poyssegur: Signal transduction pathways controlling cell proliferation; *Growth factors, clinical and therapeutical importance (J. Zapf: Clinical and therapeutic aspects of IGF-1, D.A. Fisher: The significance of EGF as a growth factor, I. Olson: Cytokines and anticytokines with special reference to tumour necrosis factor, J.W. Adamson: Erythropoietin); *Adrenals, gonads and intersexuality; *Obesity, endocrine regulation of metabolism, diabetes mellitus; D. Gupta: An integrated communication network between the immune and neuroendocrine systems in sick children; F. Delange: Endemic goiter in childhood, situation in Europe and in the world; *Calcium and bone metabolism, *Neuroendocrinology, *Growth regulation; J.E. Morley: Endocrine regulation of appetite behaviour; *Hormones and nutrition, *Pituitary and puberty, *Hormone actions – clinical and biochemical; *Andrea-Prader-Lecture:* Albert Aynsley-Green.
* Parallel sessions

Social programme:
Get-together Reception by the Governing Mayor of Berlin at the Pergamon Museum; Concert (trumpet and organ) at the Schauspielhaus, Gendarmenmarkt; Festive Banquet at Mariendorf Trotting Ground; Full day excursion to Potsdam with Sanssouci

castles and music in the park. – Accompanying persons: Sightseeing tour of the reunited Berlin; The old city; Charlottenburg Castle and Egyptian Museum; Royal Prussian Porcelain Manufacture.

Sponsors:	Deutsche Gesellschaft für Kinderheilkunde, Senat von Berlin, Ares Serono, Eli Lilly, Kabi Pharmacia-Hormones, Novo-Nordisk A/S, Berlin-Chemie, Bissendorf Peptide, Boehringer Ingelheim, Ciba Geigy, Ferring Arzneimittel, Henning Berlin, Hoechst, Hoffmann-LaRoche, Jenapharm, Mack, Merck, Milupa, Pfizer, Schering, Deutsche Wellcome.
Organising Company:	Congress Service Charité, Berlin

1992 Zaragoza	31st Annual Meeting, ESPE
Date:	6th to 9th September
Venue:	Fair Grounds (Feria de Muestras), Zaragoza, Spain
President:	Angel Ferrández Longás (E)
Secretary:	I.A. Hughes (UK)
Treasurer:	M.L. Aubert (CH)
Council:	Maité Corvol (F), S.L.S. Drop (NL), Wolfgang G. Sippell (D), N.E. Skakkebæk (DK); President- elect: I.A. Hughes (UK)
Participants (n):	600 – Reg. Fee: ESP 23,000 active, ESP 17,000 accompanying persons
Abstracts (n):	276 (53 oral, 223 poster presentations in 16 guided tours), published in Horm Res 1992;37(suppl 4):1–74

Scientific programme:
Present situation of GH therapy (J.C. Job: Report of the Working Party on hGH, M. Preece: Creutzfeldt-Jakob disease following GH treatment, N.E. Skakkebæk: Metabolic effects of GH – should GH therapy be continued in adulthood?, J.M. Wit: New therapeutic indications); Congenital hypothyroidism diagnosed by neonatal screening (J.E. Toublanc: Epidemiologic comparison of European data with those of other countries, F. Delange: Bone age studies, T. Torresani: Comparison of different methods of TSH measurement in neonatal screening, A. Grüters-Kieslich: Aetiological grouping of permanent CH with gland 'in situ', P. Rochiccioli: Mental and neurological development in CH and predictive factors); R. Blizzard: End results of paediatric endocrinopathies, H. Jacobs: Adult status of girls with gonadal-genital disorders, M. Ritzén: Adult status of boys with gonadal-genital disorders; *GH therapy, *Gonads – adrenals, *Diabetes; *Sex differentiation, *Steroids, *Gonads; Recent aspects of steroid biosynthesis in male sex differentiation (M. Zachmann: Clinical studies, M.R. Waterman:

Biochemistry and molecular biology); Fetal growth (D.J. Hill: General factors, P.D. Gluckman: Some endocrine aspects, I.K. Rossawik: Mathematical growth assessment, G. Greisen: Ultrasound and fetal growth, F. Frankenne: Human placental growth hormone); *Pituitary, *Growth – growth factors; *Genetic defects: GH – IGF, *Sex differentiation, *Adrenals; J.A. Phillips III: DNA mapping in growth and development disorders; *Andrea-Prader-Lecture:* Nathalie Josso.
* Parallel sessions
Proceedings published in Horm Res 1992;38:193–283

Social programme:
Get-together at Pignatelli Palace; Reception by the Mayor of Zaragoza at City Hall, Musical Event at Military Academy (old student music played by the 'Tuna', national dance 'Jota' of Aragón); Annual banquet at 'El Cachirulo', live music and dance; Full day excursion to Stone River Park 'Monasterio de Piedra', visit of Veruela Monastery with concert of classic and baroque music.

| Sponsors: | Ares Serono, Eli Lilly International, Kabi-Pharmacia Hormones, Novo Nordisk, Sanofi, Nestlé, Milupa, Lasa-Ipsen, Ordesa, Puleva. |

1993 San Francisco	32nd Annual Meeting, ESPE – 4th Joint Meeting with the LWPES
Date:	3rd to 7th June
Venue:	Fairmont Hotel, Stanford Court Hotel, Mark Hopkins Hotel and Masonic Auditorium, Nob Hill, San Francisco, USA
President:	Ieuan A. Hughes (UK); Melvin M. Grumbach (USA)
Secretary:	W.G. Sippell (D)
Treasurer:	M.L. Aubert (CH)
Council:	M. Corvol (F), S.L.S. Drop (NL), N.E. Skakkebæk (DK); President-elect: J.L. Van den Brande (NL)
Participants (n):	1,622 (incl. 209 students), 145 accompanying persons – Reg. Fee: USD 475 active, USD 250 students/fellows, USD 275 accompanying persons
Abstracts (n):	550 (58 oral, 492 poster presentations), published in Pediatr Res 1993;33(suppl 5):S1–S93, also lecture abstracts

Scientific programme:
Lawson-Wilkins-Lecture: Diabetes mellitus type I – islet cell destruction and growth studied in transgenic animal models (N. Sarvetnick); *T. Strachan: Molecular

pathology of 21-hydroxylase deficiency, Y. Morel: Prenatal diagnosis of CAH due to 21-OHD, S.Pang: Hormonal monitoring and side effects of prenatal dexamethasone treatment for 21-OHD CAH, M.G. Forest, H.G. Dörr: Prenatal treatment of CAH due to 21-OHD: European experience in 223 pregnancies at risk, P. Speiser: Prenatal treatment of CAH; *D. Scharp: Design and use of cellular implants for treatment of diabetes, N.K. Maclaren: Antigen directed therapies to prevent insulin dependent diabetes, A.T. Lee: Role of glucose in diabetic complications; *J. Zapf: In vivo metabolic actions of IGF-1; *R.I. Weiner: Regulation of GnRH release from GnRH neuronal cell lines, B. Franco: Kallmann syndrome – a defect in neuronal target recognition, L.W. Swanson: Spatio-temporal patterns of gene expression in the neuroendocrine system; *J. Simard: Molecular basis of CAH due to 3β-HSD deficiency, P.C. White: 11β-hydroxylase and hypertension, D.W. Russell: Steroid 5α-reductase type 2 deficiency; H.A. Ingraham: Pit-1 and its naturally occurring genetic mutations.

H.R. Bourne: G proteins in transmembrane signaling; *A.M. Spiegel: The McCune Albright syndrome – a genetically determined signal transduction disorder, U. Francke: Growth hormone insensitivity syndrome, G.I. Bell: Molecular genetics of early-onset NIDDM; *P.D. Gluckman: IGFs in normal and abnormal fetal growth, N.E. Cooke: Placental growth hormone and related proteins, D. Evain-Brion: Placental EGF receptors; *M. Trucco: Immunogenetics of type 1 diabetes mellitus, E.A.M. Gale: Population screening for risk of IDDM, C. Levy-Marchal: Incidence variation and etiology of Type 1 diabetes; *C. Carter-Su: Molecular basis of GH action, W.I. Wood: Structure and functional analysis of the hGH receptor, J.O.L. Jørgensen: GH deficiency in adulthood – effects of GH substitution; *S.H. Mellon: Neurosteroid biosynthesis: genes for adrenal steroidogenic enzymes are expressed regionally in the rat brain, S.M. Paul: Neuroactive steroids, M.D. Majewska: GABAa receptors and actions of neurosteroids; *R. Derinck: The role of TGF-β family members in mesenchymal differentiation, M.T. Corvol: Effects of 17β-estradiol on human cartilage cell proliferation and differentiation, G.E. Theintz: Bone mass growth during normal pubertal development; P.N. Goodfellow: The genetics and biochemistry of sex determination.

J.B. Gurdon: Diffusible factors and cell differentation; H. Guyda: Final height attainment in normal children with short stature treated with GH, M.B. Ranke: Height development in Turner syndrome – results of an international survey conducted by ESPE/LWPES, R.P. Kelch: Final and near final height of children with true precocious puberty treated with GnRH agonists;*C.B. Wilson: Pituitary adenomas in childhood, M.S.B. Edwards: Hypothalamic surgery and chemotherapy, S.M. Shalet: Endocrine outcome; *A.O. Brinkmann: Nuclear hormone receptors – regulators of gene expression, M.J. McPhaul: Mutations in the androgen receptor gene causing androgen resistance, J.W. Funder: Mineralocorticoid receptors; *J.G. Hall: Non-traditional forms of inheritance that are relevant for pediatric endocrinology, L.J. Shapiro: X-inactivation, E.M. Rubin: Genetically engineered mice to study endocrine disorders; *ESPE Young Investigator Award:* Jesus Argente, *Andrea-Prader-Lecture:* Martin Ritzén.

* Parallel sessions

Social programme:
Welcoming reception at Fairmont's Roof Garden; Reception at the DeYoung and Asian Art Museums in Golden Gate Park; Reception and Meeting Banquet, Fairmont Hotel; Full day excursion to Napa Valley, lunch at Inglenook Winery, return by ferry from Vallejo down San Francisco Bay.

Sponsors: Ares-Serono, Genentech, Eli Lilly & Co., Monsanto, Novo Nordisk A/S, Abbott Labs., Endocrine Sciences, Kabi Pharmacia, Ross Labs., Syntex Research, TAP Pharmaceuticals, Boots Pharmaceuticals, Bristol-Myers Squibb, Diagnostic Systems Labs., DuPont Merck, Gynex, Nichols Institute, Packard, Sandoz, Upjohn, Wyeth-Ayerst Labs.

1994 Maastricht	33rd Annual Meeting, ESPE
Date:	22nd to 25th June
Venue:	Maastricht Exhibition & Congress Centre, Maastricht, The Netherlands
President:	J. Leo Van den Brande (NL)
Secretary:	W.G. Sippell (D)
Treasurer:	S.L.S. Drop (NL)
Council:	Sergio Bernasconi (I), M. Corvol (F), Marc Maes (B), Stephen M. Shalet (UK); President-elect: A. Aynsley-Green (UK)
Participants (n):	723 active, 72 accompanying persons – Reg. Fee: NLG 500 active, NLG 325 accompanying persons
Abstracts (n):	371 (41 oral, 330 poster presentations in 29 guided tours), published in Horm Res 1994;41:45–156

Scientific programme:
P. Szolovits: Artificial intelligence, medical decision-making, and the role of the patient; D. Duboule: Hox genes and the genetic control of vertebrate limb development;

J. Baker: Postnatal phenotype of IGF-1 null mutants; *P. Czernichow: Diagnosis and treatment of diabetes insipidus, *M. Garabedian: Diagnosis and treatment of hypocalcaemia; M. Peter: Amino acid substitution R384P in aldosterone synthase causes CMO I deficiency, N.E. Skakkebæk: Expression of c-kit protooncogene protein product in gonocytes of intersex foetal and infantile testes.

J.P. Thiery: Growth factors and cell adhesion molecules as morphoregulators; T.F. Lüscher: Cell to cell communication in the blood vessel wall; D.W. Pfaff: Development of GnRH-neurons; *J. Schoemaker: Hirsutism and hyperandrogenism in adolescent girls, *F.H. Glorieux: Osteoporosis in children – a diagnostic and therapeutic challenge.T.J. Visser: Role of iodothyronine deiodinases in the regulation of thyroid

hormone bioavailability; D.R. Clemmons: IGF binding proteins and control of IGF actions; D.M. Robertson: TGF-β/inhibin family – an overview; J. Franklyn: Treatment of hyperthyrodism; *ESPE Young Investigator Award:* Peter Clayton, *Andrea-Prader-Lecture:* Maguelone Forest.
* Parallel sessions

Social programme:
Welcome reception; Concert at 'Theater aan het Vrijthof' (Netherlands Wind Ensemble); Annual Dinner at 'La Butte aux Bois', Lanaken, Belgium; Full day excursion: Limburg – Marl caves – Hoensbroek Castle. – Accompanying persons: Bus tour through the countryside, City-Walk Maastricht, Golf-clinic.

Sponsors:	Novo Nordisk, Pharmacia Kabi Peptide Hormones, Eli Lilly, Ares-Serono, Ferring, Merck, Genentech, Wyeth Laboratoria, Sandoz.
Organising Company:	Congrex Holland, Amsterdam, Netherlands

1995 Edinburgh	34th Annual Meeting, ESPE
Date:	25th to 28th June
Venue:	Edinburgh Conference Centre at Heriot-Watt University, Edinburgh, UK
President:	Albert Aynsley-Green (UK)
Secretary:	W.G. Sippell (D)
Treasurer:	S.L.S. Drop (NL)
Council:	S. Bernasconi (I), Pierre G. Chatelain (F), M. Maes (B), S.M. Shalet (UK); President-elect: C. Sultan (F)
Participants (n):	approx. 800 – Reg. Fee: GBP 280 active, GBP 180 accompanying persons, GBP 20 banquet
Abstracts (n):	404 (34 oral, 336 poster presentations, 34 read by title), published in Horm Res 1995;44(suppl 1):1–110

Scientific programme:
C.R.W. Edwards: Endocrine hypertension; *P. Donovan: Germ cell migration and development, D.C. Page: Genetic control of testis determination, M.R. Waterman: Genetic control of sex steroid synthesis; C. Sultan: Molecular genetics of androgen insensitivity; *A. Lucas: Nutritional programming, J.M. Ketelslegers: Nutritional regulation of IGF-1, S. Franks: Nutrition and reproductive endocrinology, G. Williams: Neuropeptide Y in diabetes, catabolism and exercise; P. Brickell: Hybridisation techniques, J.R.E. Davis: PCR techniques; A. Barnett: Pathogenesis of type 1 diabetes mellitus – possibilities for prediction, prevention and treatment.
   M.O. Thorner: Growth hormone secretagogues.

R.V. Thakker: Molecular endocrinology of endocrine tumours; *D.B. Dunger: The GH-IGF1 axis in IDDM, C. Kuhl: Insulin therapy: where are we now and what is the way forward?, S.S. Amiel: Studies on hypoglycaemia in IDDM, C. Levy-Marchal: The Eurodiabace project – clinical implications; *R.G. Will: Epidemiology of Creutzfeldt-Jakob disease, P. Brown: Transmissible cerebral amyloidosis and pituitary hormone therapy – an improbable connection between paediatric endocrinology and adult neurology, C. Weissmann: The role of PrP in susceptibility to prion related hormones, M. Palmer: Molecular genetics of human prion disease; A. Signore: In vivo imaging of activated lymphocytes in autoimmune disease, C.A. Hoefnagel: Scintigraphy with MIBG and somatostatin of sympathetic tumours; *ESPE Young Investigator Award:* Olaf Hiort, *Andrea-Prader-Lecture:* Pierre Sizonenko.
* Parallel sessions

Social programme:
Welcome reception at the Edinburgh Assembly Rooms; Civic reception hosted by the Lord Provost of Edinburgh at the Royal Museum of Scotland followed by a concert (Hebrides Ensemble) at the Queen's Hall; Half day excursions: The Scottish borders and Floors Castle/Whisky Galore!/The city of Edinburgh; Conference Banquet and Ceilidh at Hopetoun House, South Queensferry. – Accompanying persons: Edinburgh City – history and fashion; Glasgow and the Burrell collection.

Sponsors:	Ares Serono, City of Edinburgh District Council, Eli Lilly, Ferring, Lothian and Edinburgh Enterprise Ltd., Novo Nordisk, Pharmacia, Sandoz, Sanofi Winthrop, Scottish Convention Bureau, The WM Company, British Midland, S. Karger.
Organising Company:	Meeting Makers Ltd., Glasgow, UK

1996 Montpellier	35th Annual Meeting, ESPE
Date:	15th to 18th September
Venue:	Le Corum Conference Centre, Montpellier, France
President:	Charles Sultan (F)
Secretary:	W.G. Sippell (D)
Treasurer:	S.L.S. Drop (NL)
Council:	P.G. Chatelain (F), M. Maes (B), S.M. Shalet (UK), Raimo J. Voutilainen (FIN); President-elect: E.M. Ritzén (S)
Participants (n):	approx. 1,350 – Reg. Fee: FRF 2,500 active, FRF 300 dinner
Abstracts (n):	537 (35 oral, 451 poster presentations in 30 guided tours, 51 read by title), published in Horm Res 1996;46(suppl 2): 1–142

Scientific programme:

Pre-Congress Meeting: *International Society for Paediatric and Adolescent Diabetes (ISPAD):* Role of GH and IGF-1 in carbohydrate and lipid metabolism.

J.P. Bourguignon: Activation and inhibition of GnRH secretion, F.C.W. Wu: GnRH pulse generator during puberty in man, E. Nieschlag: Development of spermatogenesis, E.R. Simpson: Developmental aspects of aromatase expression; G. Camerino: X-linked sex reversal.

C. Junien: Genomic imprinting in paediatric endocrinology; *H.J. Anstoot: Immunology of diabetes, A. Moses: Insulin resistance, P. Czernichow: Prediction of diabetes mellitus, P.F. Bougnères: Prevention of type 1 diabetes mellitus; *I. Huhtaniemi: Role of gonadotrophins in ovarian maturation, E. Porcu: Sonographic and endocrine aspects of pubertal ovaries, G.B. Cutler: Ultrasensitive assay of plasma estradiol, R.L. Rosenfield: Polycystic ovary syndrome.

D. Mangelsdorf: Retinoids and development; *P. Aubourg: Adrenoleucodystrophy – from clinic to gene therapy, G. Chrousos: Familial glucocorticoid resistance, M. Begeot: ACTH resistance, H.G. Dörr: Adrenal insufficiency – clinical controversies; *E. Mallet: Gsα determination in pseudohypoparathyroidism, A. Spiegel: Molecular genetics of PHP, Z. Hochberg: Vitamin D resistance, R. Rizzoli: PTHrp in development and in cancer; *ESPE Research Award:* Michel Binoux, *Andrea-Prader-Prize:* Niels E. Skakkebæk.

* Parallel sessions

Social programme:

Welcome and opening ceremony, then Get-together; Champagne reception at Benedictine cloister St. Pierre, the oldest European Faculty of Medicine, then Concert at St. Pierre Cathedral; Annual dinner at Valmagne Abbey; Full day excursion to the Camargue, visit of 'La Manade Jaques Bon'. – Accompanying persons: Bus tour to the Roman city of Nîmes and Pont du Gard aquaeduct; Tour of historical city of Montpellier.

Sponsors:	Novo Nordisk, Ferring, Pharmacia & Upjohn, Eli Lilly, Ares Serono, Takeda, Sanofi-Winthrop, Ipsen, Ciba Corning, Leo, Bio Merieux.
Organising Company:	Chairman Congres, Montpellier, France

1997 Stockholm	36th Annual Meeting, ESPE – 5th Joint Meeting with the LWPES, in collaboration with APEG, JSPE and SLEP
Date:	22nd to 26th June
Venue:	Folkets Hus and Norra Latin City Conference Centre, Stockholm, Sweden
President:	Martin Ritzén (S); R.G. Rosenfeld (USA)
Secretary:	W.G. Sippell (D)
Treasurer:	S.L.S. Drop (NL)
Council:	P.G. Chatelain (F), Lourdes T. Ibanez (E), S.M. Shalet (UK), R.J. Voutilainen (FIN); President-elect: G. Giovannelli (I)
Participants (n):	1,400 active – Reg. Fee: SEK 3,200 active, SEK 2,000 fellows and East European participants, SEK 1,500 accompanying persons, SEK 200 dinner
Abstracts (n):	760 (112 oral, 760 poster in 51 guided tours, 74 of them also in 13 miniposter sessions), published in Horm Res 1997;48(suppl 2):1–201

Scientific programme:

Lawson-Wilkins-Lecture: P. Rotwein: GH receptor signalling and the nuclear actions of GH; *J.A. Gustafsson: Physiology and structure-function aspects of ERβ, D.B. Lubahn: Estrogen responses in ER- mice, F.A. Conte: Consequences of aromatase deficiency and of ER dysfunction, A. Vottero: Novel alternative splicing of P450arom mRNA in aromatase excess syndrome lymphocytes; *R. DiLauro: Genetics of thyroid development, S. Refetoff: Syndrome of resistance to thyroid hormone, J.M. DeVijlder: Defects in thyroid hormone biosynthesis, C. Reiners: Thyroid cancer – lessons from Chernobyl; *R.C. Baxter: Regulation of carbohydrate metabolism by IGFBPs, C.A. Conover: IGFBP-specific proteases, Y. Oh: IGF-independent actions of IGFBPs – new concepts for their role in growth regulation, G. Werther: Cellular localisation of IGFBPs in the rat brain following ischaemic injury; *R. Stanhope: Transfer from the paediatric endocrinologist, J.S. Christiansen: Transition of GHD patients to adult endocrinology – how and when?; *U. Ungerstedt: Microdialysis – method for steady-state studies in humans, C. Marcus: Microdialysis in paediatric endocrinology and metabolism; *L. Underwood: IGF-1 therapy – metabolic effects, D. Dunger: rhIGF-1 therapy – metabolic effects; J.M. Friedman: Leptin, leptin receptors and the control of body weight.

J. Carlstedt-Duke: Glucocorticoid receptors – structure and function; *S.A. Berenbaum: Effects of prenatal androgens on behaviour, T. Bäckström: Progestagens and CNS function, G.P. Chrousos: Effects of stress and glucocorticoids on the developing brain; *P.O. Berggren: Regulation of insulin release, H. Wallberg-Henriksson: Insulin resistance, E. Van Obberghen: Signaling through the insulin and IGF-1 receptor, M.

Murashita: Treatment with rhIGF-1 in a leprechaunism patient; *A. Wedell: Phenotype-genotype relationships in 21-OHD, W.L. Miller: Pathogenesis of lipoid CAH and the biology of StAR, K.Fujieda: StAR gene analysis in lipoid adrenal hyperplasia – functional implications, D.H. Geller: Molecular mechanism of 17,20 lyase deficiency; *Medical controversy:* *Use of hGH in normal short children (K. Albertsson-Wikland: The Swedish experience, R.L. Hintz: Final height results of the US study, J. Brämswig: 'It does not make them taller adults'); *W.G. Sippell: Many CPP children profit from treatment with GnRH agonists, G.B. Kletter: Considerations for cautious use of GnRH agonists; *Measurement of body composition (D. Bier: Non-DXA methods, C.C. Glüer: DXA and quantitative ultrasound approaches); A.H. Sinclair: New genes for boys.

D.L. Rimoin: Molecular defects in the chondrodysplasias; *P. Agre: The aquaporin family of water channels, D. Richter: ADH gene mutations, S. Nielsen: The vasopressin regulated water channel aquaporin-2; *N.E. Skakkebæk: Trends in male reproductive health – paediatric aspects, J. Mc Lachlan: Environmental hormone disruptors – occurrence and mechanisms of action, W.R. Kelce: Environmental antiandrogens – mechanisms of action; *Prenatal diagnosis and treatment of endocrine disease (S. Ratcliffe: Sex chromosome abnormalities, M.G. Forest: CAH, A. Clarke: Ethical issues, M. Holst: Scandinavian experience in CAH); *Medical Controversy:**Combined GnRHa and GH treatment (T. Tanaka: Short children with early puberty for height, T. Tuvemo: Adopted girls with precocious or early puberty, G.B. Cutler: GnRHa induced delay of epiphyseal fusion increases adult height of adolescents with short stature); *R.G. Rosenfeld: Biochemical markers of GH sensitivity, J.S. Parks: How, and how hard should we look for mutated growth genes?; *J. Müller: Management of males with 45,X/46,XY gonadal dysgenesis, C. Nihoul-Fékété: Feminising genitoplasty – when and how?; *ESPE Young Investigator Award:* Päivi Miettinen, Gerhard Binder, *ESPE Research Award Lecture:* Michel Aubert, *Andrea-Prader-Prize:* Walter Teller.
* Parallel sessions

Social programme:
Welcome reception at Norra Latin; Reception at the Stockholm City Hall (place of the Nobel prize dinner); Concert at the Royal Opera; Annual buffet dinner at Vasa Museum; Full day boat excursion through Stockholm archipelago to Vaxholm Fortress, return by bus. – Accompanying persons: Walk in the Old Town; Gripsholm Castle tour; Stockholm art tour; Drottningholm Palace tour.

Sponsors:	City of Stockholm; Pharmacia & Upjohn, Novo Nordisk, Eli Lilly, Genentech, Serono, Ferring.
Organising Company:	Congrex Sweden AB, Stockholm

1998 Florence	**37th Annual Meeting, ESPE**
Date:	24th to 27th September
Venue:	Palazzo Congressi, Florence, Italy
President:	Giorgio Giovannelli (I)
Secretary:	Martin O. Savage (UK)
Treasurer:	S.L.S. Drop (NL)
Council:	Francis E. de Zegher (B), L.T. Ibánez (E), Wieland Kiess (D), R.J. Voutilainen (FIN); President-elect: T.E. Romer (PL)
Participants (n):	1,303 active, 300 accompanying persons – Reg. Fee: ITL 600,000 active persons, ITL 70,000 Dinner
Abstracts (n):	523 (21 of symposia, 66 oral, 436 poster, 72 of them also in 12 miniposter sessions), published in Horm Res 1998; 50(suppl 3):1–150

Scientific programme:

N.K. Maclaren: New strategies for early prevention of immune mediated diabetes.

C.W. Brown: Transgenic models to study reproduction, growth and development; *P.D. Gluckman: Maternal nutritional and hormonal influences on fetal growth, F. Petraglia: Serum activin A and inhibin A levels in pregnancies complicated by IUGR, F. de Zegher: The child born small – an endocrine challenge, P. Czernichow: Reduced final height and insulin resistance in young adults born SGA; *A. Pinchera: Thyroid carcinoma in children – new perspectives, C. Giordano: Apoptosis in autoimmune thyroid diseases, G. Vassart: Non-autoimmune hyper- and hypothyroidism due to TSH receptor mutations, A. Grüters: Management of hyperthyroidism in childhood; *D. Armanini: Mineralocorticoid receptors, M.J. Dillon: Pseudohypoaldosteronism, M. Peter: Aldosterone synthase and 11β-hydroxylase deficiencies; *P. Saenger: Premature adrenarche – not always just a benign variant of puberty, L.T. Ibánez: Outcome of early hyperandrogenism in girls, B.C.J.M. Fauser: Dynamics of ovarian follicle growth throughout life, I.C.A.F. Robinson: Studies with GH secretagogues – present and future, E. Ghigo: GHRPs – state of the art and clinical perspectives.

K.A. Mahon: Genetic regulation of forebrain and pituitary development; *Current use of GH in GHD (O. Westphal: benefits, C. Volta: current challenges), Use of GH in Turner syndrome (S. de Muinck-K.-S.: benefits, Z. Hochberg: current challenges), Use of GH in short stature, IUGR and renal failure (A. Hokken-K.: benefits, P. Chatelain: cost-benefit and side effects), Misuse of GH (C. Strasburger: in sports, P. Hindmarsh: other GH misuse), New indications (W. Kiess: use of GH in catabolic states); *M. Trucco: Immunologic models of type 1 diabetes, H.B. Mortensen: Which metabolic control in children and adolescents with IDDM?, G.B. Bolli: Intensive insulin therapy and hypoglycaemia in IDDM, R. Lorini: Italian registry of young subjects at risk of developing type 1 diabetes; *ESPE Young Investigator Award:* Martin Wabitsch, *ESPE Research Award and Lecture:* Kerstin Albertsson-Wikland, *Andrea-Prader-Prize and Lecture:* Hans Åkerblom.

* Parallel sessions

Social programme:
Welcome ceremony and Get-together in the 'Salone dei Cinquecento' at Palazzo Vecchio; Organ concert in the curch of San Salvatore in Ognissanti; Gala dinner at Palazzo Corsini; Excursions (charged extra): Siena or San Gimignano or Museums of Florence. – Accompanying persons: Guided tours of Florence, Lucca or Pisa.

Sponsors:	Ares Serono, Eli Lilly, Ferring Pharmaceuticals, Novo Nordisk, Pharmacia & Upjohn.
Organising Company:	O.I.C., Florence, Italy

1999 Warsaw	38th Annual Meeting, ESPE
Date:	29th August to 1st September
Venue:	National Theatre and Opera, Warsaw, Poland
President:	Tomasz E. Romer (PL)
Secretary:	M.O. Savage (UK)
Treasurer:	W. Kiess (D)
Council:	F. de Zegher (B), L.T. Ibáñez (E), Jørn Müller (DK), Giuseppe Saggese (I); President-elect: M. Maes (B)
Participants (n):	1,207 – Reg. Fee: DEM 680 active, DEM 500 fellows and East European participants, DEM 220 accompanying persons, DEM 80 dinner
Abstracts (n):	464 (54 oral, 410 poster in 34 guided tours, 60 of them also in 10 miniposter sessions), published in Horm Res 1999; 51(suppl 2):1–153

Scientific programme:
M. Gembicki: Thyroid carcinoma related to the Chernobyl catastrophe; *Screening for congenital hypothyroidism (F. Delange: Methods for iodine deficiency screening, J.E. Toublanc: Epidemiology of CH, its relation with iodine deficiency in Eastern Europe, A. Grüters-Kieslich: Pitfalls of CH screening); *Steroid hormones and growth (N. Mauras: Androgens, G. Frank: Estrogens, O. Mehls: Glucocorticosteroids).

M. Wehling: Nongenomic action of steroids; *J. Friedman: Leptin and the regulation of body weight, W. Kiess: Hormonal regulation of circulating leptin, S. O'Rahilly: Genetic defects in human early-onset obesity; *Endocrinology of the extremely premature child (J.H. Kok: Hypothyroxinaemia, O. Söder: Postnatal growth, R. Voutilainen: Adrenal function); *Treatment of obesity in children (C.E. Flodmark: Childhood obesity and lifestyle changes achieved by psychotherapy, E. Malecka-Tendera: Pharmacological treatment); *Hirsutism at adolescence (R. Azziz: Prevalence and aetiology, L.T. Ibáñez: Diagnostic work-up and therapy); * Clinical management of CAH (W.G. Sippell, E.M. Ritzén: New aspects of 21-OHD); E. Van Obberghen: Defects of insulin action.

W.L. Miller: P450c17, adrenarche and polycystic ovary syndrome; *G. Dahlquist: Aetiology of type 1 diabetes in epidemiological perspective, M. Knip: From epidemiology to prevention, C. Boitard: Advances in immunology of diabetes; *Short stature genes (M. Dattani: Defects of hypothalamic-pituitary development, G. Rappold: SHOX mutations cause growth failure in Turner and Leri-Weill syndrome, P.E. Clayton: Defects of GH action); *Diabetes management (D. Dunger: adolescence, T. Danne: young children), *Nodular thyroid disease (A. Lewinski: Significance of preoperative cytologic examination in the diagnostics of NTD in children, T.P. Foley: Diagnostic and therapeutic approach to NTD during childhood and adolescence), *Ambiguous genitalia (I.A. Hughes: management strategy, O. Hiort: investigations); *ESPE Young Investigator Award:* Evelin Gevers, Heiko Krude, *ESPE Research Award and Lecture:* Jean-Pierre Bourguignon, *Andrea-Prader-Prize and Lecture:* Zvi Laron.
* Parallel sessions

Social programme:
Music performance and Get-together; Chopin Concert at Church of the Holy Trinity; Gala Dinner at Aula of the Technical University; Sightseeing of Warsaw or several optional tours (charged extra). – Accompanying persons: Tour of Wilanów Palace and Park; optional tours (extra).

Sponsors:	Ares-Serono, Eli Lilly, Ferring, Novo Nordisk, Pharmacia & Upjohn, Beaufour Ipsen, Intraco, Lux-Med, Novartis, Polish Ministry of Health & Welfare, Polish State Committee for Scientific Research.
Organising Company:	Congrex Sweden AB, Stockholm

2000 Brussels	39th Annual Meeting, ESPE
Date:	17th to 19th September
Venue:	Congress Centre (Palais des Congrès), Brussels, Belgium
President:	Marc Maes (B)
Secretary:	M.O. Savage (UK)
Treasurer:	W. Kiess (D)
Council:	F.E. de Zegher (B), J. Müller (DK), G. Saggese (I), Maithé Tauber (F)
Participants (n):	1,436 – Reg. Fee: EUR 390 active, EUR 200 fellows and East European participants, EUR 110 accompanying persons, EUR 60 dinner
Abstracts (n):	569 (4 plenary, 15 symposia, 45 short oral, 505 poster presentations in 135 guided discussions, 44 of them also in 8 miniposter sessions), published in Horm Res 2000; 53(suppl 2):1–191

Scientific programme:

J. Couse: ERα and ERβ knock out mouse models – relevance to human physiology and pathology; *The growth plate (B. de Combrugghe: Genetic basis of chondrocyte differentiation, J. Baron: Childhood's end – growth plate senescence and epiphyseal fusion, I.M. Shapiro: Regulation of apoptosis in cells of the growth plate), *Type 2 diabetes in childhood (F. Picard: PPARγ – a versatile metabolic regulator, A.T. Hattersley: Heterogeneity of type 2 diabetes – lessons from MODY, D.E. Hale: Epidemiological and clinical aspects).

R. Scharfmann: Control of early pancreatic development in rodent and human; ESPE Drugs and Therapeutics Committee (P. Clayton: Summary statement of GHRS on child and adolescent GHD, A. Juul: ESPE survey of diagnosis and treatment of GHD); *Mammary gland development (R.J. Santen: Hormonal regulation of the normal breast and of benign breast disease, G.D. Braunstein: Pathophysiology and management of gynecomastia, J. Russo: Developmental pattern of the human breast – implication in the susceptibility to develop benign and malignant lesions in the adult breast), *G. Van den Berghe: New insights in the neuroendocrine response to critical illness, R. Baxter: The IGF-IGFBP axis during acute and chronic illness, F. De Benedetti: Cytokines and growth impairment associated with chronic inflammation; *ESPE Research Award and Lecture:* Ze'ev Hochberg.

A. Van Steirteghem: Assisted reproductive technologies and pre-implantation genetics; *ESPE Young Investigator Award and Presentation:* Jörg Dötsch, *Andrea Prader Prize and Lecture:* Charles Brook; - *G. Saggese: Which children are at risk for osteoporosis?, E. Schönau: How to assess reliably bone structure in children?, N.J. Bishop: Are there new approaches for childhood osteoporosis?; *Interactive sessions:* *Induction of puberty in the hypogonadal girl, *Management of neonatal thyroid disorder; G.P. Chrousos: Impact of molecular biology on clinical endocrinology – past, present and future.

* Parallel sessions

Social programme:

Get-together reception at Royal Museum of Fine Arts; Bach Concert in the Cathedral of St.Michael & St.Gudule; Gala Dinner, Les Caves de Curreghem. – Accompanying persons: Half day Brussels guided tour; 3 optional tours (charged extra).

Sponsors:	Ares-Serono, Eli Lilly, Ferring, Novo Nordisk, Pharmacia & Upjohn, Beaufour-Ipsen, Henning Berlin, Karger Basel, Sabena/Swissair.
Organising Company:	Congrex Sweden AB, Stockholm

2001 Montreal	40th Annual Meeting, ESPE – 6th Joint Meeting with the LWPES, in collaboration with APEG, JSPE and SLEP
Date:	6th to 10th July
Venue:	Queen Elizabeth Hotel and Hilton Bonaventure Hotel, Montréal, Canada
President:	Guy Van Vliet (B, CDN); Harvey J. Guyda (CDN)
Secretary:	M.O. Savage (UK)
Treasurer:	W. Kiess (D)
Council:	Leo Dunkel (FIN), J. Müller (DK), G. Saggese (I), M. Tauber (F); President-elect: J. Argente (E)
Participants (n):	Over 2,000 active – Reg. Fee: CAD 675 active, CAD 375 fellows, CAD 280 accompanying persons, CAD 60 Picasso exhibition
Abstracts (n):	1,030 (9 plenary, 36 symposia, 72 short oral, 912 poster presentations), published in Pediatr Res 2001;49(6, suppl): 1A–173A

Scientific programme:

Lawson-Wilkins-Lecture: C.R. Kahn: New insights into the role of insulin in glucose homeostasis and diabetes – lessons from knockout mice; *Management of type 1 diabetes (B. Zinman: Glucose control – from conventional to intensive therapy, T.W. Jones: Hypoglycaemia risk, J.A. Edge: Causes of death), *(Mis)Perceptions of height (L.D. Voss: Short but normal – lessons from a population-based study, J.M. Wit: GH treatment and changes in QoL, D. Drotar: Models of integrating QoL factors in Pediatric clinical care), *Thyroid therapy controversies (D. Glinoer: Potential consequences of maternal hypothyroidism on the offspring, J.H. Kok: Should hypothyroxinaemic premature infants be treated?, T.P. Foley: Hyperthyroidism in children & adolescents); *J. Van den Broeck: Growth response to rhGH in TS children, F.E.de Zegher: GH treatment of SGA children, J.P. Monson: Continuing GH replacement beyond epiphyseal fusion in hypopituitarism; *G.S. Tannenbaum: Neuroregulation of GH secretion, J. Schwartz: GH signaling between receptor and nucleus, J. Baron: End organ – growth plate; *C. Polychronakos: Immunogenetics of IDDM – mechanisms of non-HLA genetic susceptibility, P. Eskelin: Molecular genetics of APCED, L.M. Mulligan: MEN; E.R.B McCabe: Mammalian sex determination – from gonads to brain.

S. Radovick: Molecular mechanisms of combined pituitary hormone deficiencies; *P.A. Boepple: Long-term outcomes after GnRH agonist therapy of girls with CPP, H. Stattin: Adult outcome of early puberty in girls, R.L. Rosenfield: Adult outcome of hyperandrogenic adolescence; *A. Larsson: Screening for CAH – costs and benefits, I.A. Hughes: CAH – optimising medical treatment, J.E.S. Jääskelainen: Sexual function and fertility in adult males and females with CAH; *R.L. Leibel: Hypothalamic regulation of energy balance, R. Strauss: Childhood obesity and self-esteem, L.H.

Epstein: Treatment of pediatric obesity; G.M. Reaven: Insulin resistance and its consequences – a major health care problem, C.H.D. Fall: Evidence for the fetal and infant origins of adult chronic disease, M.S. Kramer: Evidence against the fetal origins hypothesis of adult chronic disease; F.H. Glorieux: Osteogenesis imperfecta – new approaches to its classification and medical management.

ESPE Young Investigator Award: Ken Ong, *ESPE Research Award and Lecture:* Charles Sultan, *ESPE Outstanding Clinician Award:* Dagfinn Aarskog, *Andrea Prader Prize and Lecture:* Paul Czernichow; *R.A. Rey: Markers of testicular function in cryptorchidism, S. Schlatt: Germ cell transfer, C. Sultan: New insights into androgen action; *A. Munnich: The reality of mitochondrial medicine, R.D. Nicholls: Implications of genomic imprinting, C. Deal: Polymorphisms in the GH/IGF axis and phenotypic variability; *S. Kato: Molecular genetics of hereditary rickets, L.K. Bachrach: Assessment of bone mass, Z. Hochberg: Biology of bone maturation; A. Aynsley-Green: Hyperinsulinaemic hypoglycaemia in infancy and childhood – resolving the enigma.
* Parallel sessions

Social programme:
LWPES Welcome Reception; Erotic Picasso Exhibition at Montréal Museum of Fine Arts; Jazz Concert at Place des Arts concert hall; Optional: Laurentian mountains tour to Mont-Tremblant.

| Sponsors; Exhibitors: | Eli Lilly, Genentech, Novo Nordisk, Pharmacia, Esoterix Endocrinology, Serono; AstraZeneca, Diagnostics Systems Laboratories, Ferring, Hoffmann-La Roche, Knoll, Quest Diagnostics, Abbott, APEG, CIHR, ESPE, FHSJ, FRSQ, Grandis Biotech, IHDCYH, JSPE, S. Karger, LWPES, Merck Frosst, MiniMed, MCHF, Munksgaard, Schwarz Pharma, SLEP, Tourisme Québec, Université de Montréal. |

2002 Madrid	**41st Annual Meeting, ESPE**
Date:	25th to 28th September
Venue:	Palacio Municipal de Congresos de Madrid, Spain
President:	Jesus Argente (E)
Secretary:	M.O. Savage (UK)
Treasurer:	W. Kiess (D)
Council:	Francesco Chiarelli (I), L. Dunkel (FIN), Anita C.S. Hokken-Koelega (NL), M. Tauber (F); President-elect: C. Krzisnik (SLO)
Participants (n):	1,557 – Reg. Fee: EUR 420 active, EUR 215 fellows and East European participants, EUR 150 accompanying persons, EUR 60 gala dinner

Abstracts (n):	646 (6 plenary, 19 symposia, 45 short oral, 576 poster presentations in 49 guided tours, 40 of them also in 8 miniposter sessions), published in Horm Res 2002;58(suppl 2):1–197

Scientific programme:
J. Nerup: Genome scans and proteomics in type 1 diabetes; *J. Parks: Endocrine consequences of haploinsufficiency, P. Scambler: Molecular genetics of 22q11 deletion syndromes, B. Horsthemke: The Prader-Willi and Angelman syndromes, L.A. Pérez Jurado: Williams-Beuren syndrome; *R. Di Lauro: Genetics of congenital hypothyroidism, J. Moreno: H_2O_2 generation defects of the thyroid gland, P. Santisteban: Oncogenic mechanism of thyroid carcinomas, V.J. Pop: Maternal fT_4 levels during pregnancy and subsequent infant development – is there a critical set point of fT_4?

F.F. Casanueva: Ghrelin, a new hormone connecting growth and energy homeostasis; W.G. Sippell: Management of CAH – results of the ESPE questionnaire, E.M. Ritzén: Consensus statement on management of 21-hydroxylase deficiency, March 2002; D. Dunger: Growth, weight gain and the genetic susceptibility to TIDM and its complications, P. Czernichow: Epidemiology and clinical aspects of neonatal diabetes, J.P. Shield: The molecular basis of permanent and transient neonatal diabetes, M. Vaxillaire: Clinical and molecular spectrum of MODY; R.C. Melcangi: Neuroactive steroids regulate through growth factors the hypothalamic control of reproductive functions, S.R. Ojeda: Transgenic and genomic approaches to the study of female puberty, L.M. Garcia-Segura: Neuroprotection by sex steroids and IGF-1, R.A. Steiner: Galanin-like peptide and the integration of reproduction and body weight regulation; *ESPE Research Award and Lecture:* David Dunger.

A. Catania: α-Melanocyte-stimulating hormone; *ESPE Outstanding Clinician Award:* Jaakko Perheentupa, *ESPE Young Investigator Award Presentations:* John Achermann, Annemie Boehmer, *Andrea Prader Prize:* Jean-Louis Chaussain; J.P. Monson: Metabolic consequences of replacement and pharmacologic GH therapy, A. Lindgren: Effects of GH treatment in children with Prader-Willi syndrome, L. Hagenäs: Spontaneous growth and effects of GH treatment on height and body disproportion in achondroplasia, hypochondroplasia and dyschondrosteosis, J. Müller: GH therapy – transition from paediatric to adult care; *Interactive sessions:* *Diagnosis and treatment of the boy with delayed puberty, *Diabetes insipidus; R. Rosenfeld: Evolution and growth.
* Parallel sessions

Social programme:
Get-together reception; Classical and Flamenco Guitar Concert at Auditorio Nacional; Gala Dinner at Castillo de Viñuelas. – Accompanying persons: Half-day Madrid guided tour; museum visits, tours to Segovia or Toledo (optional).

Sponsors; Exhibitors:	Ares Serono, Eli Lilly, Ferring, Grandis Biotech, Novo Nordisk, Pharmacia; Volvo, Iberia, Freund Publishing, Ipsen Pharma, Karger, Sanofi, Wisepress, Blackwell Publishing.
Organising Company:	Congrex Sweden AB, Stockholm

2003 Ljubljana	42nd Annual Meeting, ESPE
Date:	18th to 21st September
Venue:	Cultural and Congress Centre, Ljubljana, Slovenia
President:	Ciril Krzisnik (SLO)
Secretary:	M.O. Savage (UK)
Treasurer:	W. Kiess (D)
Council:	F. Chiarelli (I), L. Dunkel (FIN), A.C.S. Hokken-Koelega (NL), M. Tauber (F); President-elect: Z. Hochberg (IL)
Participants (n):	1,381 – Reg. Fee: EUR 420 active, EUR 215 fellows and East European participants, EUR 150 accompanying persons, EUR 60 gala dinner
Abstracts (n):	592 (4 plenary, 18 symposia, 48 short oral, 522 poster presentations in 44 guided tours, 48 of them also in 8 miniposter sessions), published in Horm Res 2003;58(suppl 2):1–193

Scientific programme:
ESPE Bone Club: Treatment of osteoporosis in childhood.
S. Nielsen: Water homeostasis; *Management of precocious puberty (*interactive*), *Target cell activation (Z. Hochberg: Enzymatic modulation of glucocorticoids, L. Dunkel: Enzymatic modulation of sex steroids, J. Köhrle: Modulation of thyroid hormone availability).

R. Zorec: Molecular mechanisms of exocytosis; *ESPE Research Award and Lecture:* Annette Grüters-Kieslich; *J.L. Jameson: Congenital adrenal hypoplasia, S. Bornstein: Adrenal medulla in disorders of the adrenal cortex, C.A. Stratakis: Carney complex – molecular genetics and endocrine manifestations; *O. Hovatta: Strategies to preserve oocytes for IVF, S. Schlatt: Male germ cell transplantation, R. Ron-El: Fertility in Klinefelter syndrome.

M. Holzenberger: IGF-1 and longevity; *ESPE Outstanding Clinician Award:* Otto Westphal, *ESPE Young Investigator Award:* Delphine Jaquet, José Moreno, *Andrea Prader Prize:* Michael Ranke; *Permanent cure for diabetes (L. Falqui: Pancreatic islet transplantation and prospects of gene therapy, I.R. Cohen: Immunologic intervention in T-cell mediated destruction of beta cells, F.R. Kaufman: Glucose sensors and the promise of a closed-loop system; *U. Kuhnle: Intersexuality – medicine, nature and culture?, H. Meyer-Bahlburg: Long-term psychological outcome of children born with

uncertain sex, P. Ransley: Dilemmas and responsibilities in intersex management – the role of the surgeon; *H. Werner: IGF-1, IGF receptors and overgrowth, C. Gicquel: Assessment of patients referred for overgrowth syndrome, L.G. Biesecker: Manifestations of Proteus syndrome – a disorder of mosaic overgrowth; P. Cohen: The GH-IGF system and cancer risk.
* Parallel sessions

Social programme:
Opening ceremony with concert and welcome reception, reception for new ESPE members, professors and participants of ESPE Summer and Winter Schools; Afternoon excursion to Postojna caves with concert of 'Camerata Labacensis'; Gala Dinner at Grand Hotel Union followed by live music and dancing. – Accompanying persons: City tour of Ljubljana; Tour to Bled or to the Adriatic Sea (optional).

Sponsors; Exhibitors:	Eli Lilly, Ferring, Novo Nordisk, Pfizer, Sandoz, Serono; ESPE, Ipsen, Karger, Sanofi-Synthelabo, Serono Symposia International Foundation, Society for Endocrinology & Bioscientifica
Organising Company:	Congrex Sweden AB, Stockholm

2004 Basel	43rd Annual Meeting, ESPE
Date:	10th to 13th September
Venue:	Messe Basel, Switzerland
President:	Ze'ev Hochberg (IL)
Secretary:	M.O. Savage (UK)
Treasurer:	W. Kiess (D)
Council:	Jean-Claude Carel (F), P. Czernichow (F), Sabine De Muinck Keizer-Schrama (NL), Peter C. Hindmarsh (UK), A. Hokken-Koelega (NL), Olof Söder (S); Secretary-elect: F. Chiarelli (I), President-elect: Y. Morel (F)
Participants (n):	1,694 – Reg. Fee: EUR 410 active, EUR 215 fellows and East European participants, EUR 100 accompanying persons, EUR 45 party
Abstracts (n):	652 (12 plenary, 32 symposia/'Meet the Expert', 71 short oral/'Clinical Focus', 537 poster presentations – no guided tours, no miniposter sessions), published in Horm Res 2004;62(suppl 2):1–215

Scientific programme:
ESPE Bone Club: Neonatal bone and mineral; *2 Satellite Symposia.*

R. Zinkernagel: Immunoprotection – immunopathology – autoimmunity? J.F. Bach: Immunotherapy of type-1 diabetes; *M.A. Levine: The rachitic bone, M.K. Drezner: Hypophosphataemic rickets, T.D. Thacher: Calcium deficiency rickets; *Endocrinology of the acutely ill child (H. Soreq: Inherited and acquired parameters in stress and anxiety responses, G. Chrousos: HPA axis and critical illness, A.C.S. Hokken-Koelega: Early endocrine predictors of outcome; *M.O. Savage: Growth failure in chronic inflammatory disease; *Z. Zadik: Diagnosis of GHD; *M. Polak: Diabetes in the very young child; *M.A. Levine: Childhood osteoporosis; *J.C. Carel: Indications for GnRH therapy; E. Nevo: Evolution and stress, U. Schibler: The mammalian circadian timing system; *2 Satellite Symposia.

J.Å. Gustafsson: New paradigms in estrogen signaling and their clinical implications, W.F. Crowley: Genes controlling the onset and maintenance of reproductive function in the human; *ESPE Research Award and Lecture:* Francis de Zegher, *ESPE Outstanding Clinician Award:* Emanuele Cacciari; *D.J. Waxman: Mechanisms in the pulsatility of GH signaling, S.J. Frank: Generation of GHBP and modulation of cellular GH sensitivity, C.J. Strasburger: Treatment with long-acting GH; *K.L. Parker: Ovarian development, P.G. Crosignani: Amenorrhea – diagnosis and management, D. Apter: Contraception during adolescence; *L. Sävendahl: Actions of sex steroids on the growth plate, P.C. Hindmarsh: Sexual dimorphism in intrauterine and infantile growth, D.B. Dunger: Sexual dimorphism in body composition; *Yearbook Session 1;* *Workshop:* Building a clinical trial.

P. Bianco: Skeletal stem cells – physiology and disease, K. Skorecki: Insulin producing human embryonic stem cells; *ESPE Young Investigator Award:* Taneli Raivio, *Andrea Prader Prize:* Steven Shalet; *G. Reach: Theoretical basis of glucose monitoring, T. Danne: Continuous s.c. glucose monitoring in children, T.H. Koschinsky: Glucose monitoring systems in the future; *S. Mandrup: Regulation of adipocyte differentiation and function, I.S. Farooqi: Genetics of severe childhood obesity, M.C.J. Rudolf: International consensus development on childhood obesity; *H. Cedar: Basic mechanisms of imprinting, G.E. Moore: Genomic imprinting in fetal growth restriction, H. Jüppner: PHP – a spectrum of imprinted disorders caused by GNAS mutations; *A.E. Dunaif: PCOS, *Yearbook Session 2;* *New technologies (K. Pacak: PET in the evaluation of endocrine tumours, C. Sultan: Ultra-sensitive determination of serum estrogen and androgen bioactivity in children); *ESPE Hormone Research Prize:* Sylvie Tenoutasse; A. Cama: Molecular mechanisms of insulin resistance, A.E. Dunaif: Insulin resistance and reproduction in PCOS.

* Parallel sessions

Social programme:

Get-together; Concert at Stadt-Casino (Moran Children Choir, Israel); Welcome reception for new ESPE members and their sponsors, ESPE party. – Accompanying persons: Tour of Old Basel; Lucerne and the Swiss alpes (including rack-railway to top of Mt. Pilatus); Visit of Beyeler Foundation museum of modern art, cruise on the Rhine (optional).

Sponsors; Exhibitors: Eli Lilly, Ferring, Ipsen, Novo Nordisk, Pfizer, Sandoz, Serono; Astra Zeneca, ESPE, Freund Publishing, Karger, Oxford Bio-Innovation, Sanofi-Synthelabo, Serono Symposia, Wisepress, 3w-informed.

Organising Company: Congrex Sweden AB, Stockholm

2005 Lyon	**44th Annual Meeting, ESPE – 7th Joint Meeting with the LWPES, in collaboration with APEG, APPES, JSPE and SLEP**
Date:	21st to 24th September
Venue:	Lyon Convention Centre, Lyon, France
President:	Yves Morel (F)
Secretary General:	Francesco Chiarelli (I)
Council:	W. Kiess (D), chair FC; Z. Hochberg (IL), chair POC; S.L.S. Drop (NL), chair ETC, President-elect; Stefano Cianfarani (I), chair CPC; J.C. Carel (F); O. Söder (S)
Participants (n):	3,146 – Reg. Fee: EUR 410 active members, EUR 550 non-members, EUR 215 fellows and East European participants, EUR 100 accompanying persons, EUR 69 dinner
Abstracts (n):	1,371 (11 plenary, 47 symposia, 90 short oral, 1223 poster presentations, 73 of them also in 12 miniposter sessions), published in Horm Res 2005;64(suppl 1):1–429.

Scientific programme:

ESPE Bone Club: Diagnosis and treatment of genetic bone disorders; *ESPE Yearbook Session; Business Meetings (*5 Societies); *5 Satellite Symposia.

6 Meet the Expert(MTE) Seminars (M. Phillip: Modern Delivery of insulin, S. Rivkees: Radioactive iodine and Graves' disease, M. Rivarola: The infant with ambiguous genitalia, I. Arnhold: Investigation of the short child, H. Tanaka: Congenital bone diseases, H. Storr: Investigation of Cushing syndrome); *Lawson-Wilkins-Lecture:* S.R. Ojeda: The mystery of mammalian puberty – how much more do we know?; *C. Sultan: Clinical expression of PCO, S. Franks: Pathophysiology and genetics of PCO, P. Vuguin: Treatment of PCO; *S. Amselem: Hypothalamic-pituitary development, M. Maghnie: Modern imaging of developmental anomalies of the pituitary, R. Pfäffle: Genotype-phenotype correlations; *M. Waters: Insights into GH receptor function, S. Yakar: Animal models of IGF-1 deficiency, P. Bougnères: GH receptor exon 3 polymorphism and variations of skeletal growth; *L. Ward: Osteoporosis in children due to chronic illness – etiology and diagnosis, L.K. Bachrach: – treatment and monitoring, Z. Hochberg: Rickets in the Middle East; *S. Refetoff: Neurological and thyroid abnormalities, G. Francis: Management and outcome of children with differentiated thyroid cancer, M. Polak: Management of fetus and infant of the mother with Graves' disease; W.L. Miller: Understanding steroid physiology by studying rare diseases; *3 Satellite Symposia.

ESPE Hormone Research Prize: Lonneke De Boer; Y. Matsuzawa: Adipocytokines and obesity-related diseases; *César- Bergadá-Lecture:* A.C. Latronico: LH and FSH receptor mutations; *ISPAD-ESPE-LWPES Symposium (A. Schmidt: Receptor for advanced glycation endproducts and vascular complications of diabetes, D. Daneman: Prevention and treatment of diabetic nephropathy, D. Dunger: Modulation of the GH-IGF axis); *P. de Lonlay: Molecular basis of hyperinsulinism, T. Otonkoski: Imaging techniques, C. Stanley: Management of neonatal hyperinsulinism; *K. Fujieda: Transcription factors and adrenal development, A. Clark: New causes of primary adrenal insufficiency, M.G. Forest: Prenatal treatment of CAH due to 21-OHD – update of French multicentre study; *N. de Roux: New genetic defects in the control of pubertal onset, L. Dunkel: Gonadal function in Klinefelter syndrome, G. Conway: Premature ovarian failure; *N. Mauras: Nutritional benefits of GH and testosterone treatment, C. Camacho-Hübner: IGF-1 treatment, D. Simon: GH treatment in corticosteroid-treated children; Global inequalities in paediatric endocrine care (P. Gluckman: Interventions to improve fetal growth, M. Silink: Improving diabetes care, A. Grüters-Kieslich: Paediatric thyroid diseases, P. Raghupathy: Growth surveillance and consequences of impaired nutrition, M. Savage & F. Cassorla: Statement of minimal acceptable care); *3 Satellite Symposia.

ESPE Young Investigator Award: Christa Flück, *Outstanding Clinician Award:* Jean-Claude Job, *Research Award and Lecture:* Serge Amselem, *Andrea Prader Prize:* Wolfgang Sippell; *C. Levy-Marchal: Obesity, insulin resistance and metabolic syndrome, S. Caprio: Metabolic phenotype of prediabetes, S.A. Arslanian: Prevention and treatment of type 2 diabetes in youth; *R. Rosenfeld: Deconstruction of idiopathic short stature, C. Quigley: GH increases final height in ISS – results of a randomised, placebo-controlled trial, J.M. Wit: ISS – GH dose effect with and without inhibition of puberty, D. Sandberg: Psychological aspects of short stature; *E. Vilain: Mechanisms of gonadal differentiation, B.B. Mendonca: Spectrum of intersex – aetiology and phenotype, G. Warne: Long term outcome of the intersex child; *L. de Lacerda: Genetics, clinical presentation and treatment of adrenal tumours, P. Niccoli-Sire: Investigation and management of MEN, M.B. Barontini: Familial pheochromocytoma, C. Sklar: Endocrine consequences of cancer treatment; *F. Cucca: Genetic and autoimmune mechanisms of type 1 diabetes, P. Eskelin: Polyglandular autoimmune syndrome, J.C. Carel: Proinsulin as an autoimmune target; J. Samarut: Thyroid hormone receptors.
* Parallel sessions

Social programme:
Welcome reception; Lyon Gourmet Dinner at Halle Tony Garnier. – Accompanying persons: Tour of Old Lyon; Lyon, the silk capital (walking tour); Tour to the Beaujolais region (extra).

Sponsors; Exhibitors:	Eli Lilly, Ferring, Genentech, Ipsen, Novo Nordisk, Pfizer, Sandoz, Serono; AACE, Astra Zeneca, Bayer Healthcare, DSL, ESPE, Freund Publ., Immunodiagnostic Systems, IPWSO, Karger, LWPES, Medtronic, Sanofi-Aventis, Serono Symposia, Stratec, Tercica, Valera, Wisepress, World Sci. Publ., 3W-Informed.
Organising Company:	Congrex Sweden AB, Stockholm

2006 Rotterdam	45th Annual Meeting, ESPE
Date:	30th June to 3rd July
Venue:	De Doelen Concert and Congress Centre, Rotterdam, The Netherlands
President:	Stenvert L.S. Drop (NL)
Secretary General:	F. Chiarelli (I)
Council:	O. Söder (S), chair FC; S. Cianfarani (I), chair CPC; Z. Hochberg (IL), chair POC; J.C. Carel (F), chair Summer School; R. Voutilainen (FIN), President-elect.
Participants (n):	1,869 – Reg. Fee: EUR 400 active members, EUR 600 non-members, EUR 225 fellows and East European participants, EUR 100 accompanying persons, EUR 40 dinner
Abstracts (n):	654 (7 plenary, 31 symposia/'New technology', 74 short oral/'Clinical Focus', 542 poster presentations in 46 guided tours), published in Horm Res 2006;65(suppl 4):1–213

Scientific programme:
ESPE Bone Club: Skeletal complications of chronic systemic diseases; *ESPE Growth Plate WG:* Multidisciplinary approach to growth plate biology; *ESPE Obesity Club:* Pathophysiology of childhood obesity; *ESPE WG on Turner Syndrome:* TS morbidity and prevention; *Workshop: Diabetes 2006 – Global issues, global challenges; 1 Satellite Symposium.

The Dawn of Aging (J. Hoeijmakers: DNA damage repair, cancer, aging and life span extension, S.W.J. Lamberts: Aging and the IGF system; *Update Consensus Meetings: Disorders of sex development / Management of the SGA child; *D. LeRoith: Clinical relevance of systemic and local IGF-1 and IGFBPs, C. Cowell: Auxologic indices for GH therapy – Australian experience, K. Albertsson-Wikland: Prediction of GH treatment response; *A.G. Uitterlinden: Genetic influence on bone mass and fracture risk in paediatric patients, N. Bishop: Treatment modalities in paediatric bone disease, E. Schönau: Mechanography – quantitative analysis of muscle function; *A. Plagemann: Perinatal programming of the orexigenic system, D. Marks: Melanocortin signaling in obesity and cachexia, S. Farooqi: Role of genetic factors in childhood obesity;

*S. Bornstein: Cytokines and their effects on steroidogenesis, inflammation and the HPA axis, L. Sävendahl: Cytokine effect on growth plate chondrocytes, S.F. Ahmed: Promoting growth in children with chronic disease; *2 Satellite Symposia.

S. Obici: How the hypothalamus controls glucose production, E. van Cauter: Endocrinology of sleep; *ESPE Young Investigator Award:* Mireille Castanet, *Research Award and Lecture:* Mikael Knip; *6 Meet the Expert(MTE) Seminars (S. DeMuinck K-S: Turner puberty induction, C.L. Acerini: Detection of early microvascular complications in IDDM children, J. Gregory: Neonatal hypoglycaemia, M. Polak: Hypothyroidism, C. Sultan: GnRH independent precocious puberty, P. Mullis: Genetic forms of hypopituitarism); *Interactive session* (P.C. Sizonenko: To menstruate or not, that is the question!, A. Richter-Unruh: Two boys with precocious puberty); *New technology* (M. Benson: Clinical implications of systems biology and high-throughput technology in paediatrics, E. Clynen: Proteomics in endocrine research and practice); *ESPE Yearbook Session 1; 1 Satellite Symposium.

B. Roep: Immunopathogenesis of diabetes mellitus type 1, A. Hattersley: Low birth weight and type 2 diabetes – fetal programming or shared genes; *ESPE Outstanding Clinician Award:* Ruth Illig, *Andrea Prader Prize:* Ieuan Hughes; *W. Arlt: Pre-receptor regulation of steroid hormones, C.L. Smith: Clinical implications of steroid receptor coactivators, S. Lajic: Long-term effects of prenatal glucocorticoid treatment in CAH (*ESPE Research Unit Lecture*); *ESPE/ISPAD Symposium* (M. Knip: Primary prevention of diabetes: cow milk, sunlight, vitamins and other interventions, M. Hummel: Delaying exposure to wheat and barley proteins to reduce diabetes incidence, P. Pozzilli: Prevention of diabetes in children); *Endocrine disrupters (R.M. Sharpe: Development of male reproductive system – targets for phthalates and other EDs, J. Toppari: Trends in congenital abnormalities of MRS – possible role of EDs, K.M. Main: EDs in breast milk and alteration; *Interactive session* (J. Lebl: A girl with hypertension, C.L. Deal: Adiposity – it's all in the family!); *New technology* (S.A. Wudy: GC-MS profiling of steroids in times of molecular biology, C. Knopf: Steroid metabolomics using GC-MS); *ESPE Yearbook Session 2; *ESPE Hormone Research Prize:* Paul-Martin Holterhus; Kári Stefánsson: Population genomics and paediatric endocrinology.
* Parallel sessions

Social programme:
Welcome reception; Concert by the Rotterdam Chamber Orchestra, followed by ESPE Evening (dinner, music, dancing). – Accompanying persons: Rotterdam museum tour; Half day visit to Delft (Blue pottery, Nieuwe Kerk); Extra: Full day tour of Rotterdam (by boat) and Gouda.

Sponsors; Exhibitors:	Eli Lilly, Ferring, Ipsen, Novo Nordisk, Pfizer Endocrine Care, Sandoz, Serono; Astra Zeneca, Demeditec Diagnostics, ESPE, IGEA, IPWSO, Karger, LWPES/ESPE 2009, Medtronic, Serono Symposia, Stratec Med, Tercica, Valera, Wisepress.
Organising Company:	Congrex Sweden AB, Stockholm

2007 Helsinki	**46th Annual Meeting, ESPE**
Date:	27th to 30th June
Venue:	The Helsinki Fair Centre, Helsinki, Finland
President:	Raimo J. Voutilainen (FIN)
Secretary General:	F. Chiarelli (I)
Council:	O. Söder (S), chair FC; S. Cianfarani (I), chair CPC; S.L.S. Drop (NL), chair ETC; Z. Hochberg (IL), chair POC; Christopher J.H. Kelnar (UK), chair CLB; Juliane Léger (F); A. Büyükgebiz (TR), President-elect.
Participants (n):	2,302
Abstracts (n):	742 (9 plenary, 40 symposia/'Research Methods', 90 short oral/'Working Groups', 603 poster presentations – no guided tours), published in Horm Res 2007;68(suppl 1):1–282

Scientific programme:
ESPE Growth Plate WG: Multidisciplinary approach to growth plate biology; *ESPE Obesity Club:* Management of juvenile morbid obesity; *ESPE Turner Syndrome WG:* Puberty induction and hormonal replacement therapy; *ESPE Bone Club:* New diagnostics and treatment of paediatric bone disease; *Workshop Diabetes 2007:* Paediatric endocrinology and diabetes in Africa, *ESPE Yearbook Session 1; *2 Satellite Symposia.*

*Basic research (D. Kelberman: SOX2 is expressed in forebrain and pituitary during human embryonic development, E. Charmandari: LBD of hGRα confers transactivation, R. Miclea: Loss of apc inhibits osteo- and chondrogenic differentiation); *6 Meet the Expert(MTE) Seminars* (L. Dunkel: Treatment of male HH, T. Battelino: Intensive insulin therapy, J. Achermann: Diagnosing the newborn with DSD, N. Shaw: Treatment of childhood osteoporosis, H. Krude: Treatment of hyperthyreosis, J. Perheentupa: Treatment of APECED in practice); U. Pagotto: Endocannabinoid system in endocrine regulation and energy balance, P. Gluckman: Can fetal programming after IUGR be reversed postnatally?; *Research Methods 1* (W.J. Gerver: Short-term effects of GH on body composition as a predictor for growth, R. Pfäffle: Evaluating the effects of mutations); *ESPE/ISPAD Symposium* (A. Ziegler: Risk factors for β-cell autoimmunity in offspring of affected parents, O. Simell: From genetic susceptibility to clinical disease, M. Revers: Evidence for gene-environmental interactions?; *Cryptorchidism (I.A. Hughes: Genetic and endocrine regulation of testicular descent, J. Hutson: Hormones or knives?, M. Ritzén: Optimal age for treatment?); *Craniopharyngioma (R. Buslei: Classification, G. Nikkhah: Stereotactic treatment, R. Lustig: Hypothalamic obesity – mechanisms and management); Perinatal endocrinology (S. Franks: Fetal origins of PCOS, K. Watterberg: HPA function and glucocorticoid treatment in extremely premature newborns); *2 Satellite Symposia.*

*Clinical research (A. Abulibdeh: Neonatal onset of AR familial neurohypophyseal DI, T. Raivio: FGF8 is a key ligand for FGFR1 in GnRH ontogeny, C. Camacho-Hübner: Severe GH insensitivity in siblings due to a Stat5b gene defect is associated with 2 distinct immune disorders); P. Ross: Mechanism of osteoclastic bone resorption, K. Alitalo: Lymphangiogenesis in development and human disease; *Research Methods 2 (P. Jüni: Case control studies, P. Lichtenstein: Twin studies); *Autoimmune polyendocrinopathy (J. Perheentupa: Disease phenotype, L. Peltonen: Mutations and pathophysiology, A. Liston: Modulation of immune pathologies in Aire KO mice by genetic manipulation of organ susceptibility); *Lipids (S. Gidding: PDAY study – origins of atherosclerosis, H. Niinikoski: 15 year dietary intervention study STRIP, A. Wiegmann: Medical treatment of hyperlipidemia); *Preterm infants' growth (Z. Hochberg: Evolutionary perspectives of infantile growth, J.M. Wit: Growth restraint, D.Dunger: Insulin therapy in preterm newborns); *ESPE Yearbook Session 2; *Ethics of GH treatment of short stature (K. Albertsson-Wikland: Pro treatment, E. Malecka-Tendera: Controversies and unsolved problems); *ESPE Young Investigator Award:* Antje Körner, *Research Award and Lecture:* Primus Mullis; *2 Satellite Symposia.

ESPE Outstanding Clinician Award: Cathérine Dacou-Voutetakis, *Hormone Research Prize:* Burak Salgin, Sandrine Ostermann, *Andrea Prader Prize:* Martin Savage; *Management of subclinical hypothyroidism (P. Mullis: Pro, A. Grüters-Kieslich: Contra treatment); *A. Tiulpakov: Screening and characterisation of DAX-1 interacting proteins *(Research Unit Lecture)*, M. Phillip: Consensus meeting report: Continuous insulin infusion treatment up-date; *D. Eizirik: Targets for prevention of β-cell death in type 1 diabetes, S. Bonner-Weir: β-cell regeneration as therapeutic option for treatment of insulin deficiency?, J.C. Henquin: In vitro deregulation ofinsulin secretion in infantile hyperinsulinism; *Monogenic growth disorders (M. Lipsanen-Nyman: Mulibrey nanism, O. Mäkitie: Cartilage hair hypoplasia, M.L. Warmann: Short stature due to mutations in NPR2); K. Ong: Looking for candidate genes in complex diseases.
* Parallel session

Social programme:
Welcome reception at Helsinki City Hall; ESPE Evening at Hilton Kalastajatorppa hotel with dinner and midsummernight dancing; ESPE Nordic walking (4 km), start at Olympic stadium (Nurmi statue). – Accompanying persons: Full day excursion to Old Town of Porvoo; Conducted tour of Suomenlinna sea fortress.

Sponsors; Exhibitors:	Eli Lilly, Ferring, Ipsen, Merck Serono, Novo Nordisk, Pfizer Endocrine Care, Sandoz; Astra Zeneca, Beammed-Sunlight, ESPE, Freund Publ., IPWSO, ISPAD 2007, LWPES/ESPE 2009, Medtronic, Phoenix Europe, Karger, Serono Symposia, Wisepress.
Organising Company:	Congrex Sweden AB, Stockholm

2008 Istanbul	**47th Annual Meeting, ESPE**
Date:	20th to 23rd September
Venue:	Lüfti Kirdar Convention Centre (ICEC), Istanbul, Turkey
President:	Atilla Büyükgebiz (TR)
Secretary General:	F. Chiarelli (I), President-elect
Council:	O. Söder (S), chair FC; S. Cianfarani (I), chair CPC; Moshe Phillip (IL), chair ETC; Jean-Claude Carel (F), chair POC; C.J.H. Kelnar (UK), chair CLB; J. Léger (F).
Participants (n):	2,841
Abstracts (n):	750 (10 plenary, 34 symposia/'New technologies', 108 short oral/'Working Groups', 598 poster presentations – no guided tours), published in Horm Res 2008;70(suppl 1):1–281

Scientific programme:
*Joint Session, ESPE Bone Club & ESPE Growth Plate WG; *ESPE Turner Syndrome WG:* TS and the cardiovascular system; *ESPE Obesity Club:* Metabolic syndrome in the paediatric age range; *ESPE DSD WG:* European activities and research on DSD; – *ESPE-ISPAD Symposium:* A cure for diabetes (T. Battelino: Closed loop insulin delivery, P. de Vos: Insulin-producing stem cells, A. Secchi: Pancreas and islet transplantation); *Hyperandrogenism in adolescent girls (M. Pugeat: Physiopathology of androgen synthesis and action in women, M.L. Anttila: Genetics of PCOS, F. Kelestimur: Differential diagnosis and treatment); *P. Gluckman: Human evolution and the timing of puberty, G. Chrousos: Evolution of steroid hormone receptors, M. Wallis: Evolution of GH and prolactin; *Istanbul – bridge the gap in child health* (T. Turmen: Health status of children between East and West, X. Luo: Providing endocrine care in a large country, A. Virmani: Poverty as a confounding factor); – E. Jablonka: Epigenetic inheritance, G. Hotamishgil: The growing pandemic of obesity and associated chronic diseases; *2 Satellite Symposia.*

From Gene to Disease (M. Rassoulzadegan: RNA-mediated epigenetic heredity, P.O. Berggren: Signal transduction in type 1 diabetes; *7 Meet the Expert(MTE) Seminars* (N. Güngör: Type 2 DM, E.Malecka-Tendera: Management of obesity, H. Spoudeas: Endocrine management of cancer survivors, L. Ibañez: Hirsutism and menstrual disturbances, M. Tauber: Prader-Willi syndrome, J. Argente: Delayed puberty, N. Kandemir: Interpretation of endocrine tests); *ESPE Yearbook Session 1; *New technologies 1* (A. Krook: Gene silencing, R. Loos: Genes for obesity and related traits); *Interactive session 1* (A. Körner: Faces of the brain, F. Mahmud: Failure to GH therapy); *2 Satellite Symposia.*

ESPE Young Investigator Award: Luisa de Sanctis, *Research Award and Lecture:* Leo Dunkel; *JSPE/ESPE Plenary Lecture:* T. Ogata: DSD – new genes and new mechanisms; S. Bulun: Sexual differentiation, development and behaviour – lessons from aromatase mutations; *Interactive session 2* (S. Drop: 2 patients with tall stature, J. Brämswig: The myth of multiple endocrinopathies); *B. Koletzko: Early feeding and child obesity, S. Ozanne: Long term metabolic consequences of early malnutrition, A. Singhal: Long term consequences of feeding premature infants; *S. Grosse: Prevention of intellectual disability by CH newborn screening – quantitation, G. Van Vliet: – in industrialised contries, H. Krude: - in developing countries; *S. Amselem: Genetic networks and child growth, S. Ojeda: Searching for upper-echelon genes controlling female puberty, R. Scharfmann: Genetic networks and islet development; J. Majzoub: Central water and electrolyte homeostasis, S. Nielsen: The aquaporin water channel; *2 Satellite Symposia.*

ESPE Outstanding Clinician Award: Ferenc Péter, *Andrea Prader Prize:* Stenvert Drop; *J.M. Wit: Idiopathic short stature, J.C. Carel: Use of GnRH agonists in children, M. Karperien: Genome-wide expression analysis of human chondrocytes *(Research Unit Lecture);* *C. Reiners: Radiation induced thyroid cancer in children, A. Pinchera: Clinical approach to thyroid nodules, B. Jarzab: Molecular profile of thyroid tumours; *P. Ducy: Endocrine regulation of energy metabolism by the skeleton, M. Schülke: Regulation of muscle mass by novel endocrine factors and by mechano-endocrine coupling, D. Vesley: Novel cardiovascular hormones; *ESPE Yearbook Session 2;* *New technologies 2* (M.J. Santiago: New imaging PET, L. Hertz-Pannier: Brain, development and hormones – new MR techniques).
* Parallel session

Social programme:
Welcome reception at ICEC; ESPE Evening and dinner at 1001 Column Cistern. – Accompanying persons: Istanbul grand tour (full day).

Sponsors, Exhibitors:	Eli Lilly, Ferring, Ipsen, Merck Serono, Novo Nordisk, Pfizer Endocrine Care, Sandoz; Animas, BioGlobe, Biopartners, Biospace, ESPE, Gentest, Genzyme, IPWSO, Johnson& Johnson, LWPES/ESPE 2009, Medtronic, Probiz, Karger, Serono Symposia.
Organising Company:	Congrex Sweden AB, Stockholm

2009 New York	**48th Annual Meeting, ESPE – 8th Joint Meeting with the LWPES, in collaboration with APEG, APPES, JSPE and SLEP**
Date:	9th to 12th September
Venue:	Hilton New York, N.Y., USA
President:	Paul Saenger (USA); Francesco Chiarelli (I)
Secretary General:	F. Chiarelli (I)
Council:	O. Söder (S), chair FC; J.C. Carel (F), chair POC; S. Cianfarani (I), chair CPC; C.J.H. Kelnar (UK), chair CLB; J. Léger (F); Moshe Phillip (IL), chair ETC; Jan Lebl (CZ), President-elect.
Participants (n):	more than 3,600
Abstracts (n):	1,329 (14 plenary, 53 symposia, 108 free communications, 14 'Clubs/ Working Groups', 1251 poster presentations, 78 read by title), published in Horm Res 2009;72(suppl 3):1–547

Scientific programme:
3 Club Sessions: *Bone/Growth Plate/Turner S., *DSD Working Group, *Obesity Club: Epigenetics of childhood obesity; *Yearbook Session 1, *Endocrinology of Malnutrition; *3 Satellite Symposia*.

15 Meet the Expert(MTE) Sessions; C. Junien: Early and lifelong remodelling of our epigenomes by nutrition, D.G. Bichet: Aquaporin channel disorders and clinical implications; *Yearbook Session 2;* *Adrenarche revisited (R.J. Auchus: Molecular basis, S. Wudy: Clinical implications of premature adrenarche, B.J.Ellis: Family relationships); *P.E. Cryer: Hypoglycemia, functional brain failure and death, D. Daneman: Prevention of hypoglycemia in children, J. Zonszein: Hypoglycemia a conundrum; *J.P. Bourguignon: Assessment of pubertal timing, A.C. Latronico: New mutations in abnormal puberty, A.B. Migliano: Natural selection and age of first reproduction in pygmy populations; *Endocrine pathology of the premature infant (G. Van Vliet: Screening for thyroid disorders, V. Mericq: Nutrient enhanced formula effects on insulin sensitivity and body composition, R. Voutilainen: Adrenal function; *Prolactin (G. Vincent: New biology concepts, H.R. Boquete: Hyperprolactinemia, A. Beckers: Epidemiology of prolactinomas); *ESPE Hormone Research Prize:* Eric Mallet, Klaus Mohnike, *Outstanding Clinician Award:* Giuseppe Chiumello, *Andrea Prader Prize:* Jan-Maarten Wit; - *2 Satellite Symposia*.

*6 MTE Sessions, *Yearbook Session 3; - M.J. Waters: The GH receptor – update on mechanism and actions, H.M. Domené: Human ALS deficiency; *Endocrine imaging (L.J. States: Congenital hyperinsulinism, J.A. Carrasquillo: Adrenals, M. Maghnie: Anterior pituitary); *ISPAD-Symposium:* P.S. Zeitler: Type 2 diabetes – TODAY study at baseline, F.R. Kaufman: The HEALTHY trial, M. Knip: Update on Finnish trials;

*Longevity (M. Holzenberger: Insulin/IGF-1 signaling in the mouse, P. Cohen: GH/IGF system in human longevity, M.O. Thorner: Longevity versus healthspan); *I.C.A.F. Robinson: A journey up and down the GH/IGF-1 axis; - *A. Virmani: Type 2 diabetes in South Asians, W.C. Knowler: Diabetes in American Indian populations, E.A. Davis: Type 2 diabetes in indigenous Australian children; *Genome wide association screening (J.N. Hirschhorn: GWAS for pediatric endocrinology, M.R. Palmert: Investigating variation in pubertal timing, R.J.F. Loos: Obesity-related traits, S.C.L. Gough: Autoimmune thyroid disease); *Sex chromosomes (J.A.M. Graves: Weird animal genomes and human sex chromosomes, L. Carrel: Gene expression from the inactive X, G.A. Rappold: SHOX and disease); *Pro/Con Sessions (T. H. Inge – M. Wabitsch: Pediatric bariatric surgery; M. Freemark – T. Hannon: Insulin sensitizers); *Vitamin D biology (D. Goltzman: Genetic mouse models, V. Bhatia: Mother-child vitamin D deficiency, T.O. Carpenter: FGF23, vitamin D and bone); – S. Kato: Biology and function of nuclear steroid hormone receptors, A.M. Spiegel: Inherited endocrine diseases involving G proteins and – receptors; - *Satellite Symposium.*

8 MTE Sessions; ESPE Research Award and Lecture: Yves Le Bouc, *ESPE Young Investigator Award:* Felix Riepe; - S.F. Ahmed: European DSD register; A.A.L. Joge *(SLEP)*: Isolated SHOX haploinsufficiency; - *Molecular basis of adrenal disorders (J.C. Achermann: Transcriptional regulation of adrenal development, W.L. Miller: P450 oxidoreductase deficiency, T. Tajima: Classic and nonclassic lipoid CAH, C.A. Stratakis: Adrenal tumorigenesis); *Syndromic DSD (T. Ogata: Genetic causes of hypospadias, E. Vilain: Hormones and genes in sex development, C. Bouvattier: Long term follow-up of DSD patients); *Bone biology (F. Rauch: Skeletal development in children, D.G. Little: Manipulation of mechanisms in bone repair); *Insulin resistance in children (C. Levy-Marchal: Consensus conference results, S. Arslanian: Risk factors and consequences, A. Sinaiko: Methods for measurement and screening); - J.A. Todd: Genome-wide genetic profiling of type1 diabetes – but what next?, P.E. Scherer: Adiponectin.

* Parallel session

Social programme:
Welcome Reception; President's Poster Symposium / Reception.

Sponsors:
Eli Lilly, Genentech, Ipsen/Tercica, Merck Serono, Novo Nordisk, Pfizer, Sandoz, Teva.

2010 Prague	**49th Annual Meeting, ESPE**
Date:	22nd to 25th September
Venue:	Prague Congress Centre (PCC), Prague, Czech Republic
President:	Jan Lebl (CZ)
Secretary General:	F. Chiarelli (I)
Council:	O. Söder (S), chair FSC; J.C. Carel (F), chair POC; S. Cianfarani (I), chair CPC; M. Phillip (IL), chair ETC; Gary Butler (UK); Feyza Darendiler (TR); C.J.H. Kelnar (UK), chair CLB and President-elect.
Participants (n):	3,205
Abstracts (n):	1001 (9 plenary, 37 symposia/'new perspectives', 84 free communications, 29 working groups, 712 poster presentations, 130 read by title), published in Horm Res Paediatr 2010; 74(suppl 3):1–316

Scientific programme:

5 Working Group sessions: *New discoveries in bone and growth plate physiology; *European DSD registry/management of testicular DSD; *Development of adipose tissue in children; *Adolescent PCOS; *Brain morphology and function in Turner syndrome/care of TS girls questionnaire; - O. Cinek: Autoimmune polyendocrine syndrome type 1; *Ovarian development (M. Fellous: FOXL2 and downstream events, A. Biason-Lauber: WnT4 and R-spondin 1 signaling, K. McElreavey: NR5A1(SF1) and premature ovarian failure); *Diabetes immunotherapy (C. Boitard: Mechanisms and targets of intervention, J. Ludvigsson: Immunomodulation with GAD, K.C. Herold: Anti-CD3 therapy); *IGFs and nervous system (M. Holzenberger: Brain IGF-1 receptors control growth and lifespan, A. Musarò: IGF-1 in neuromuscular disease, D. Ley: IGF-1 as protector of brain and vessel development in preterm infants); *4 MTE sessions; 3 Satellite Symposia.*

Yearbook Session 1; *Towards the future cure of diabetes (M. Phillip: Closing the loop, O. Kelly: Macroencapsulated beta cells from embryonic stem cells); J.C. Brüning: How the fetal hypothalamus senses maternal glucose metabolism, G. Karsenty: The crosstalk bone – energy metabolism); *ESPE Young Investigator Award:* Martine Cools, *Hormone Research Prize:* Talia Eldar-Geva, Jerzy Starzyk, *ESPE Research Award and Lecture:* Peter Clayton; *Adrenals – *ESPE/SLEP* (A. Hübner: Triple A syndrome, A.C. Latronico: Adrenocortical carcinomas and p53 mutations, W. Arlt: PAPSS2 deficiency and adrenal hyperandrogenism); *Environmental endocrine disruption (R. Sharpe: The masculinisation programming window, M. Skinner: Transgenerational actions of EDs – epigenetic ghosts in your genome, J. Toppari: Human implications); *The SWEET project –*ESPE/ISPAD* (Z. Šumnik: Heterogeneity of paediatric diabetes care in Europe, C. De Beaufort: Standards for centres of reference, T. Danne: Role of IT); *4 MTE sessions; 2 Satellite Symposia.*

Yearbook Session 2; *New treatment modalities for preservation of fertility (S. Schlatt: Testicular stem cells, M. Rosendahl: Girls and women facing gonadotoxic treatment); *ESPE Outstanding Clinician Award:* Herwig Frisch, *Andrea Prader Prize:* Ze'ev Hochberg; - *Beta cell (A.T. Hattersley: Potassium channel mutations and diabetes, P.R. Njølstad: Carboxyl ester lipase and diabetes, O. Rubio-Cabezas: Diabetes due to neurogenin 3 deficiency); *Epigenetics (M. Constância: Introduction, K.A. Lillycrop: Nutrition, epigenetics and developmental plasticity, L.H. Lumey: Changes after prenatal exposure to Dutch famine 1944-45); *Puberty (N. Pitteloud: Genetics of IHH, K. Ong: Common genetic variants and timing of puberty, A. Juul: Secular trends in Europe – environmental factors); G. Vassart: Specificity and promiscuity of G-protein coupled receptors, T. Tajima *(K. Fujieda memorial lecture)*: Molecular basis of adrenal insufficiency); *1 Satellite Symposium.*

Yearbook Session 3; *Thyroid (H. Krude: Thyroid dysgenesis and movement disturbance – NKX2.1, J. Moreno: Iodide recycling defects – DEHAL1, T. Visser: Severe developmental delay and thyroid hormone transport – MCT8); *DSD management (M. Hines: Gender identity in DSD patients, D.F. Swaab: Sexual differentiation of the human brain, P. Mouriquand: Impact on surgical management); – J.S. Parks: PROP1 and the bridge to Krk.

* Parallel session

Social programme:
Welcome reception; ESPE Evening at Žofin Palace (live music, dinner and dancing). – Accompanying persons: Grand Tour of Prague; optional sightseeing tours: Old town and Jewish quarters; Český Krumlov; Baroque Prague.

Sponsors; Exhibitors:	Eli Lilly, Ferring, Ipsen, Merck Serono, Novo Nordisk, Pfizer Endocrine Care, Sandoz; Demeditec Diagnostics, ESPE, ESPE 2011, IPWSO, ISPAD, PerkinElmer, Karger, Serono Symposia, Society for Endocrinology, European Paediatric Association, Visiana Aps, Wisepress.
Organising Company:	Congrex Sweden AB, Stockholm

2011 Glasgow	**50th Annual Meeting, ESPE**
Date:	25th to 28th September
Venue:	Scottish Exhibition and Conference Centre, Glasgow, UK
President:	Christopher J.H. Kelnar (GB)
Secretary General:	F. Chiarelli (I)
Council:	O. Söder (S), chair FSC; J.C. Carel (F), chair POC; S. Cianfarani (I), chair CPC; C.J.H. Kelnar (GB), chair CLB; M. Phillip (IL), chair ETC; Gary Butler (GB); Feyza Darendiler (TR); W. Kiess (D), President-elect.

Participants (n):   over 3,500 expected – Reg. Fee: EUR 460 member, EUR 660 non-member, EUR 285 fellows, retired etc., EUR 95 accompanying persons, EUR 95 ESPE evening

Abstracts (n):   published in Horm Res Paediatr 2011;76(suppl 2)

Scientific programme:
Evidence-based Paediatric Endocrinology – its strengths and limitations

5 Working Group Sessions: *ESPE Bone and Growth Plate Working Group; *ESPE DSD Working Group (European collaborative activities; Issues in etiology and management of testicular DSD); *ESPE Obesity Working Group: Long and short-term consequences of childhood obesity; *ESPE Paediatric and Adolescent Gynaecology Working Group: Amenorrhea in adolescence; *ESPE Turner syndrome Working Group: Ovarian failure in TS.

Sir I. Chalmers: The research community needs to serve the information needs of patients and professionals more effectively, M. Bland: Improving statistical quality in published research; *Evidence-based medicine in growth assessment – in memory of Prof. J. Tanner (J.L. Baker: How to define thinness, overweight and obesity in children at population level, G. Butler: Can we replace national growth charts with WHO growth standards?, S. van Buuren: Evidence-based screening for short stature); *Early life origins of health and disease (C. Levy-Marchal: Effect of in utero and early-life conditions on adult health and disease, R. Simmons: Epigenetic regulation of beta-cell function in fetal growth retardation, J. Seckl: Prenatal stress, glucocorticoids and the programming of adult disease); *New insights in phosphate metabolism (Z. Hochberg: Deciphering hypophosphataemic rickets, D. Prié: FGF23 in health and disease, H. Jüppner: Genetic control of phosphate metabolism); *4 MTE sessions;*2 Satellite Symposia.

*4 MTE sessions; *New perspectives in brain imaging (J. Haynes: Decoding mental states from human brain activity, K. Simmons: Using fMRI to map conceptual representations of food and reward), *Yearbook session 1; Frontiers in diabetes (B. Cannon: Is brown adipose tissue changing our metabolic world?, Å. Lernmark: Immune therapy in type 1 diabetes); *ESPE Awards & Activities 1;* *Principles of evidence-based medicine (M. Offringa: Not just small adults – the need for high quality trial evidence in children, R.L. Smyth: Ensuring safe and effective medicines for children, R. Gilbert: Educating the educators), *Long term safety of drugs in children (P. Laurberg: Concern with long term tolerance of thyroid hormone replacement?, J.C. Marini: Bisphosphonates – proceed with caution, M. Hero: Aromatase inhibitors and sex steroids), *Unexpected effects of hormones on the brain (A. Sirigu: How oxytocin affects human brain and behaviour, M. Schumacher: Neuroprotective actions of progesterone, O. Baud: Melatonin and neuroprotection), *4 MTE sessions;*2 Satellite Symposia.

*4 MTE sessions; *New perspectives in molecular analysis (C. Ruivenkamp: CGH arrays, I. Netchine: DNA methylation techniques), *Yearbook session 2; ESPE Awards & Activities 2; *ISPAD/ESPE Symposium (W. Tamborlane: Sensor augmented pump therapy, E. Gale: Evidence and guidelines in diabetes treatment, R.W. Holl: Gathering evidence for diabetes treatment from large databases), *Cortisol-cortisone shuttle (P.M. Stewart: 11β-HSD mutations and the HPA axis, B.R. Walker: 11β-HSD1 inhibitors for metabolic syndrome and beyond, J.R. Challis: Adverse effects of maternal glucocorticoids – role of the 11β-HSD placental barrier), *Impact of chronic conditions on growth (F. De Luca: Impaired growth plate chondrogenesis in children with chronic illnesses, F. De Benedetti: Impact of chronic inflammation on the growing skeleton, B. Bailleul: Nutritional signals, somatotropic axis, and lifespan); I. Barroso: Exome analysis and the future of molecular medicine; *2 Satellite Symposia.

*Yearbook session 3; *Evidence-based medicine in thyroid diseases (A. van Wassenaer: Prophylactic postnatal thyroid hormones for morbidity and mortality prevention in preterm infants, S. Rivkees: Graves' disease – management controversies and options, F. De Luca: Subclinical hypothyroidism), *Pathogenesis of PCOS – APPES/ESPE Symposium (D.H. Abbott: Transient in utero androgen excess and glucose intolerance – lessons from animal models, Z-J. Chen: Genetic factors in PCOS – new insights from China, F. Cassorla: Reproductive function of women with PCOS), *GH long term safety (L. Robison: GH exposure – results from the childhood cancer survivor study, J-C. Carel: Long-term mortality after rGH for Isolated childhood short stature – the French SAGhE study, L. Sävendahl: SAGhE update, E. Abadie: Review of GH products by EMA); Food for thought before going home (G. Chrousos: The evolution of homeostasis and stress mechanisms, T. Tanaka (*ESPE/JSPE Lecture*): Growth promoting therapies in short children at onset of puberty – an evidence-based appraisal).
* Parallel session

Social programme:
Welcome Reception at Glasgow Science Centre; ESPE Evening: '50th Birthday Party' including the ESPE Benefit Concert for the Children of Japan, given by the Chamber Orchestra of Europe, then Ceilidh (dinner, music and dance). – Accompanying persons: Tours of Glasgow and countryside.

Sponsors; Exhibitors:	Eli Lilly, Ferring, Ipsen, Merck Serono, Novo Nordisk, Pfizer Endocrine Care, Sandoz; Dutch Growth and Research Foundation, Enobia Pharma, European Pediatric Association, ESPE 2012 Leipzig, ESPE, IPWSO, ISPAD, Karger, PC PAL, Serono Symposia International Foundation, Turner Syndrome Support Society, Visiana Aps, Wisepress
Organising Company:	Congrex Sweden AB, Stockholm

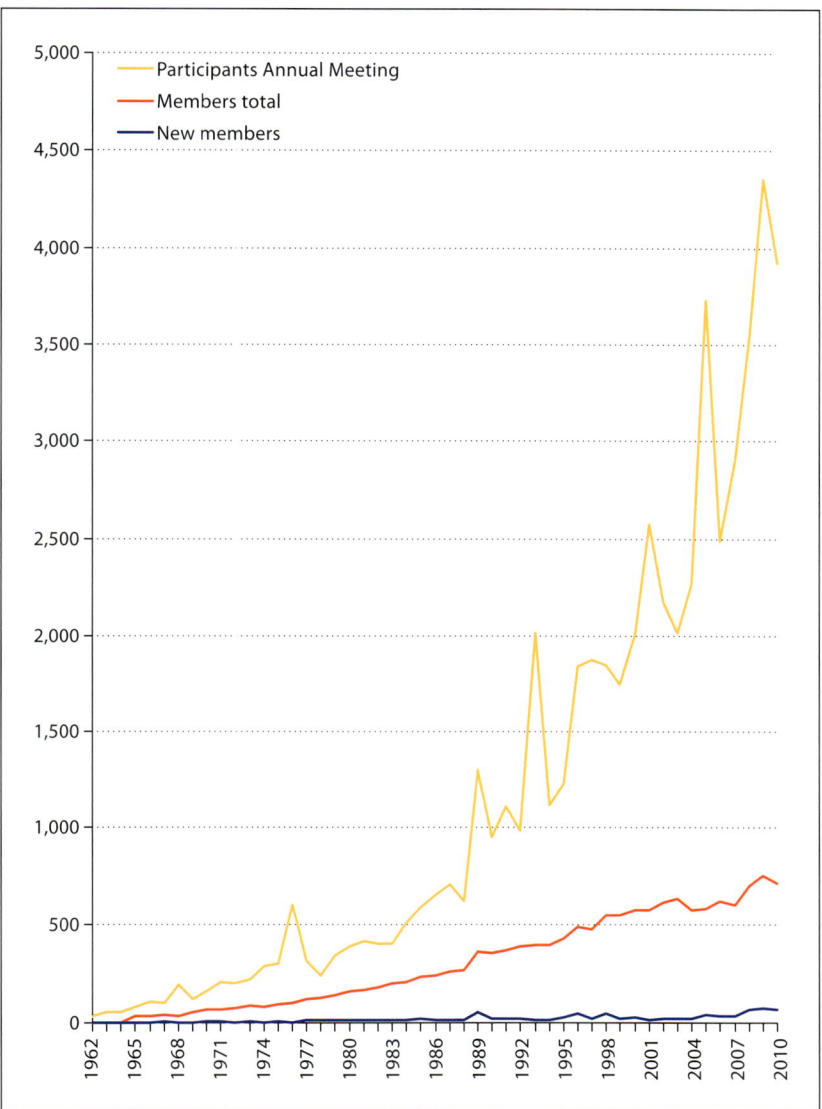

Graph showing development of ESPE members and participants at the annual meetings. Note that ESPE membership appears to grow in a linear fashion, in contrast to the exponential growth in the number of participants at the annual meetings.

Secretaries, Treasurers and Honorary Members

ESPE Secretaries

1965–1971	Henk Visser
1971–1977	Milo Zachmann
1977–1982	Ralph Rappaport
1982–1987	Albert Aynsley-Green
1987–1992	Ieuan Hughes
1992–1997	Wolfgang Sippell
1997–2004	Martin Savage
2004–2011	Franco Chiarelli
2011–	Lars Sävendahl

ESPE Treasurers

1965–1971	Henk Visser
1971–1977	Leo Van den Brande
1977–1983	Pierre Sizonenko
1983–1993	Michel Aubert
1993–1998	Sten Drop
1998–2005	Wieland Kiess
2005–2011	Olle Söder

ESPE Honorary Members

1968	Douglas Hubble (died 1981)
1995	Andrea Prader (died 2001)
1997	James (Jim) Tanner (died 2010)
1998	Dietrich (Dieter) Knorr
2002	Hendrick (Henk) Visser

EUROPEAN SOCIETY FOR PAEDIATRIC ENDOCRINOLOGY

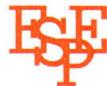

Professor Dr. med. Andrea Prader

is elected as

HONORARY MEMBER

to the

EUROPEAN SOCIETY FOR PAEDIATRIC ENDOCRINOLOGY

by the ESPE Business Meeting held on the occasion of the 34th Annual Meeting
in recognition of his outstanding contribution to paediatric endocrinology and of his role in
the founding of this Society

EDINBURGH, 25th JUNE 1995

Albert Aynsley-Green
ESPE President

Wolfgang G. Sippell
ESPE Secretary

Stenvert L.S. Drop
ESPE Treasurer

Charles Sultan
ESPE President-Elect

Sergio Bernasconi
ESPE Council

Pierre Chatelain
ESPE Council

Marc Maes
ESPE Council

Stephen M. Shalet
ESPE Council

ESPE Schools

Summer School

Sponsored by Ferring Pharmaceuticals A/S for the benefit of young paediatric endocrinologists in training in ESPE countries.

For 3 days, usually preceding the Annual Meeting, an international faculty of about 15 teachers and 25 students selected by the ESPE Summer School Steering Committee deal with three different areas from the field of paediatric endocrinology. Teachers lecture on their specialist subject and students present case reports to illustrate the chosen topics. In-depth discussions, within and outside the programme, help establish contact between younger and older paediatric endocrinologists and among future ESPE members. The programme is organised by the ESPE Summer School Steering Committee.

Fellows who have successfully attended the Summer School will be entitled to 1 year's free ESPE membership (conditions apply and will be notified during attendance of the Summer School).

Date	Venue	Coordinator	Topics		
1987	Chateau de Bonas, Toulouse, France	Dr. Paul Czernichow	growth and growth factors	perinatal growth and energy expenditure	intersex
1988	Liselund, Slagelse, Denmark	Dr. Leo Van den Brande	puberty	thyroid	diabetes
1989	Kibbutz Nof Ginosar, Israel	Dr. Leo Van den Brande	growth factors	diabetic retinopathy and nephropathy	vasopressin and diabetes insipidus

Date	Venue	Coordinator	Topics			
1990	Burg Feistritz, Vienna, Austria	Dr. Pierre Sizonenko	calcium, vitamin D and PTH	sexual differentiation	sports and endocrinology	
1991	Alkersum, Föhr Island, Germany	Dr. Pierre Sizonenko	female genital system	diabetes insipidus	thyroid hormone	
1992	Jaca, Pyrenees, Spain	Dr. Pierre Sizonenko	adrenal	the renin-angiotensin system	peptide hormones	endocrine sequelae of tumour therapy
1993	Asilomar, California, USA	Dr. Pierre Sizonenko	puberty	carbohydrate metabolism	hormone-binding proteins	
1994	Engelenburg, Arnhem, The Netherlands	Dr. Martin Savage	neuroendocrinology	sexual differentiation	Insulin secretion and action	
1995	Blairquhan Castle, Glasgow, UK	Dr. Martin Savage	calcium	thyroid disorders	aspects of puberty	
1996	Duché d'Uzès, Nimes, France	Dr. Martin Savage	adrenal gland	endocrine control of fluid balance	the GH-IGF1 axis	
1997	Roslagens Pärla, Ljusterö, Sweden	Dr. Martin Savage	reproductive physiology	carbohydrate metabolism	endocrinopathy of chronic illness	
1998	Cartusia Pontiniani, Siena, Italy	Dr. Maguelone Forest	sex differentiation	neurological aspects of obesity and appetite	bone metabolism	Turner syndrome
1999	Kazimierz Dolny, Poland	Dr. Maguelone Forest	puberty	perinatal endocrinology	aspects of growth	
2000	Castel-des Sorbiers, Belgium	Dr. Maguelone Forest	aspects of overgrowth	type 1 diabetes	environment and endocrine systems	screening for endocrine disorders
2001	Manoir Alpine, Ste-Adèle, Quebec, Canada	Dr. Maguelone Forest	hormone resistance	puberty	oncology	molecular basis of endocrine diseases

Date	Venue	Coordinator	Topics			
2002	Parador Hotel, Segovia, Spain	Dr. Annette Grüters-Kieslich	pituitary development and disorders	vitamin D, calcium and PTH	disorders of male sexual differentiation	obesity and type 2 diabetes
2003	Grand Hotel Toplice, Bled, Slovenia	Dr. Annette Grüters-Kieslich	diabetes insipidus	hypoglycaemia	diabetes mellitus	congenital adrenal hyperplasia
2004	Bad Ramsach, Switzerland	Dr. Annette Grüters-Kieslich	steroid receptors	precocious and delayed puberty	growth hormone insensitivity	
2005	Annecy, France	Dr. Annette Grüters-Kieslich	congenital hypothyroidism	adrenal disorders	insulin resistance	paediatric bone disorders
2006	Nunspeet, Netherlands	Dr. Jean-Claude Carel	imaging	male undermasculinisation	tumours in paediatric endocrinology	issues in growth hormone therapy
2007	Helsinki, Finland	Dr. Jean-Claude Carel	type 1 diabetes	polygenic heritability	calcium disorders	ovarian function
2008	Sapanca, Turkey	Dr. Lars Sävendahl	hyperthyroidism and thyroid nodules	abnormal pubertal development	skeletal dysplasias and rickets	
2009	Briarcliff Manor, New York, USA	Dr. Lars Sävendahl	disorders of sexual development (DSD)	obesity, type 2 diabetes, metabolic syndrome	endocrine manifestations of cancer	auto-immunity
2010	Sychrov, Czech Republic	Dr. Lars Sävendahl	neuroendocrinology	puberty	type 1 diabetes mellitus	nutritional effects on bone physiology
2011	Auchen Castle, UK	Dr. Faisal Ahmed	growth	thyroid	disorders of sex development	type 1 diabetes mellitus

Winter School

The ESPE Winter School was modelled on the Summer School and, with the opening up of Eastern Europe, was established with the support of Ferring Arzneimittel, Kiel, for the benefit of young paediatric endocrinologists from those European and Mediterranean countries where training in this field is not adequate in the home situation.

For one week, an international faculty of teachers, tutors and students deal with aspects of basic training in paediatric endocrinology. Through lectures, group work sessions and case presentations, students are enabled to participate actively and successfully at ESPE meetings and in the various programmes. The programme is organized by the ESPE Winter School Steering Committee.

Date	Venue	Coordinator
1995	Seregélyes, Hungary	Dr. Ze'ev Hochberg
1997	Lezno, Poland	Dr. Ze'ev Hochberg
1998	Bistritza, Bulgaria	Dr. Ze'ev Hochberg
1999	Moscow, Russia	Dr. Henriette Delemarre-Van de Waal
2000	Prague, Czech Republic	Dr. Henriette Delemarre-Van de Waal
2001	Bucharest, Romania	Dr. Henriette Delemarre-Van de Waal
2002	Izmir, Turkey	Dr. Jørn Müller
2003	Minsk, Belarus	Dr. Angela Hübner
2004	Vilnius, Lithuania	Dr. Angela Hübner
2005	Dobógokö, Hungary	Dr. Angela Hübner
2006	Varna, Bulgaria	Dr. Angela Hübner
2007	Prague, Czech Republic	Dr. Angela Hübner
2008	Ain Soukhna, Egypt	Dr. Malcolm Donaldson
2009	Moscow, Russia	Dr. Malcolm Donaldson
2010	Dareddaya, Morocco	Dr. Malcolm Donaldson
2011	Ankara, Turkey	Dr. Malcolm Donaldson

Committees and Working Groups

ESPE Council Committees and the Chairs in June 2011

Clinical Practice Committee (Chairman: Dr. Gary Butler, London, UK)
The Clinical Practice Committee compiles and maintains a list of drugs/therapeutic agents (including agents/drugs used for investigation) relevant to the practice of Paediatric Endocrinology throughout Europe.

Education and Training Committee (ETC) (Chairman: Dr. Jan Lebl, Prague, Czech Republic)
The Training Committee has the objective of promoting the training and education of young paediatric endocrinologists throughout the world.

Finance and Strategic Committee (Chairman: Dr. Olle Söder, Stockholm, Sweden)
The mission of the Finance and Strategic Committee is to advise the Council on financial strategy and resources, to monitor investments, income and expenditure and to administer the financial aspects of grants and fellowships.

Programme Organising Committee (POC) (Chairman: Dr. Jean-Claude Carel, Paris, France)
The Programme Organising Committee (POC) is responsible for organising the programme of the Society's annual meeting.

Other ESPE Committees

Andrea Prader Committee (Chair: Dr. Franco Chiarelli, Chieti, Italy)
Clinical Fellowship Committee (Chair: Dr. Chris Kelnar, Edinburgh, UK)
Newsletter Editorial Board (Chair: Dr. Jesús Argente, Madrid, Spain)
Research Fellowship Committee (Chair: Dr. Jesús Argente; Madrid, Spain)
Research Unit Advisory Panel (Chair: Dr. Irène Netchine, Paris, France)

Sabbatical Leave Programme Committee (Chair: Dr. Jan-Maarten Wit, Leiden, The Netherlands)
Summer School Steering Committee (Chair: Dr. Faisal Ahmed, Glasgow, UK)
Winter School Steering Committee (Chair: Dr. Malcolm Donaldson, Glasgow, UK)
Travel Grant Steering Committee (Chair: Dr. Franco Chiarelli, Chieti, Italy; Dr. Olle Söder, Stockholm, Sweden)
Web Editorial Board (Chair: Dr. Gary Butler, London, UK)
Visiting Scholarship (Chair: Dr. Franco Chiarelli, Chieti, Italy)

ESPE Working Groups

ESPE Bone and Growth Plate Working Group
ESPE DSD (Disorders of Sexual Differentiation) Working Group
ESPE Obesity Working Group
ESPE Turner Syndrome Working Group
ESPE PAG (Paediatric and Adolescent Gynaecology) Working Group

ESPE Facts

Consensus Statements

Organisational (policy) principles to guide and standardise the child health care system and/or improve the health of children with endocrine disease in Europe.

To collect information, discuss improvements, and indicate ideal or just acceptable paths for the management of the child with endocrine diseases.

1998	ESPE/GRS: Consensus guidelines for the diagnosis and treatment of adults with growth hormone deficiency: summary statement of the Growth Hormone Research Society Workshop on Adult Growth Hormone Deficiency. J Clin Endocrinol Metab 1998;83:379–381	
2000	ESPE/GRS: Consensus guidelines for the diagnosis and treatment of growth hormone (GH) deficiency in childhood and adolescence: summary statement of the GH Research Society. J Clin Endocrinol Metab 2000;85:3990–3993	
2002	ESPE/LWPES CAH Working Group: Consensus statement on 21-hydroxylase deficiency. Horm Res 2002;58:188-195/J Clin Endocrinol Metab 2002;87:4048–4053	
2003	ESPE (Drugs and Therapeutics Committee): Growth hormone treatment and risk of solid tumours. Horm Res 2003;60:103–104	
2004	ESPE/LWPES: Consensus Statement on diabetic ketoacidosis in children and adolescents. Arch Dis Child 2004;89:188–194/Pediatrics 2004;113: 133–140	
2004	ESPE Working Group on Congenital Hypothyroidism: Guidelines for neonatal screening programs for congenital hypothyroidism. Horm Res 1994;41:1–2	
2005	Consensus statement on minimal acceptable care in paediatric endocrinology. Horm Res 2006;65:111–113.	
2005	Consensus statement on the management of the GH-treated adolescent in the transition to adult care. Eur J Endocrinol 2005;152:165–170	
2006	ESPE/LWPES: Consensus statement on management of intersex disorders. Arch Dis Child 2006;91:554–563	

2007	ESPE/GRS/LWPES/JES/ESA: Consensus guidelines for the diagnosis and treatment of adults with GH deficiency. Eur J Endocrinol 2007;157: 695–700
2007	Management of the child born small for gestational age through to adulthood: a consensus statement of the International Societies of Pediatric Endocrinology and GRS. J Clin Endocrinol Metab 2007;92: 804–810
2007	ESPE/LWPES/ISPAD, endorsed by ADA and EASD: Consensus Statement: use of insulin pump therapy in the pediatric age-group. Diabetes Care 2007;30:1653–1662
2008	GRS/LWPES/ESPE: Consensus Statement on the Diagnosis and Treatment of Children with Idiopathic Short Stature. J Clin Endocrinol Metab 2008;93:4210–4217
2009	ESPE/LWPES: Consensus statement on the use of GnRH analogs in children. Pediatrics 2009;123:752–762
2010	ESPE/LWPES/ISPAD/APPES/APEG/SLEP/JSPE: Insulin resistance in children: consensus, perspective, and future directions. J Clin Endocrinol Metab 2010;95:5189–5198
2011 (planned)	ESPE/LWPES/ISPAD: Consensus statement on the use of continuous glucose sensors (CGS) in the paediatric age group

Awards and Scholarships

Andrea Prader Prize

This prize was established with the support of Pharmacia, Stockholm (now Pfizer), as Leadership Award given to a member of the Society in recognition of achievements within the field of paediatric endocrinology. It was named after ESPE's founding father and was first awarded in 1988.

The winner is selected by the Andrea Prader Prize Committee, which meets especially for this purpose. The committee is chaired by the ESPE Secretary and includes a renowned endocrinologist who is not a member of ESPE.

Previous Winners		
1988	Dr. Milo Zachmann	Zurich, Switzerland
1989	Dr. Leo Van den Brande	Utrecht, The Netherlands
1990	Dr. Raphael Rappaport	Paris, France
1991	Dr. Albert Aynsley-Green	Newcastle upon Tyne, UK
1992	Dr. Nathalie Josso	Montrouge, France
1993	Dr. Martin Ritzèn	Stockholm, Sweden
1994	Dr. Maguelone Forest	Lyon, France
1995	Dr. Pierre Sizonenko	Geneva, Switzerland
1996	Dr. Niels Skakkebaek	Copenhagen, Denmark
1997	Dr. Walter Teller	Ulm, Germany
1998	Dr. Hans Åkerblom	Helsinki, Finland
1999	Dr. Zvi Laron	Petah Tikva, Israel
2000	Dr. Charles Brook	London, UK
2001	Dr. Paul Czernichow	Paris, France
2002	Dr. Jean-Louis Chaussain	Paris, France
2003	Dr. Michael Ranke	Tübingen, Germany
2004	Dr. Stephen Shalet	Manchester, UK
2005	Dr. Wolfgang G. Sippell	Kiel, Germany
2006	Dr. Ieuan Hughes	Cambridge, UK
2007	Dr. Martin Savage	London, UK
2008	Dr. Stenvert Drop	Rotterdam, The Netherlands

Previous Winners		
2009	Dr. Jan Maarten Wit	Leiden, The Netherlands
2010	Dr. Ze'ev Hochberg	Haifa, Israel
2011	Dr. Charles Sultan	Montpellier, France

ESPE Research Award

This award was established in 1996, with the sponsorship of Pharmacia, Stockholm (now Pfizer).

It is given to an ESPE member in recognition of research achievements of outstanding quality in the fields of basic endocrine science or clinical paediatric endocrinology. The prize is awarded through nomination and selection by the Andrea Prader Prize Committee.

Previous Winners		
1996	Dr. Michel Binoux	Paris, France
1997	Dr. Michel Aubert	Geneva, Switzerland
1998	Dr. Kerstin Albertsson-Wikland	Gothenburg, Sweden
1999	Dr. Jean-Pierre, Bourguignon	Liège, Belgium
2000	Dr. Ze'ev Hochberg	Haifa, Israel
2001	Dr. Charles Sultan	Montpellier, France
2002	Dr. David Dunger	Cambridge, UK
2003	Dr. Annette Grüters-Kieslich	Berlin, Germany
2004	Dr. Francis de Zegher	Leuven, Belgium
2005	Dr. Serge Amselem	Creteil, France
2006	Dr. Mikael Knip	Helsinki, Finland
2007	Dr. Primus Mullis	Bern, Switzerland
2008	Dr. Leo Dunkel	Kuopio, Finland
2009	Dr. Yves Le Bouc	Paris, France
2010	Dr. Peter Clayton	Manchester, UK
2011	Dr. Anita Hokken-Koelega	Rotterdam, The Netherlands

ESPE Young Investigator Award

This award was established in 1993 with the sponsorship of Pharmacia, Stockholm (now Pfizer). It is conferred to a young practising European paediatrician, not older than 40 years of age by the end of the year in which the Award is given, in recognition of his/her scientific publications.

Previous Winners		
1993	Dr. Jesus Argente	Madrid, Spain
1994	Dr. Peter Clayton	Manchester, UK
1995	Dr. Olaf Hiort	Lübeck, Germany
1996	Not awarded	
1997	Dr. Päivi J Miettinen	Helsinki, Finland
	Dr. Gerhard Binder	Tübingen, Germany
1998	Dr. Martin Wabitsch	Ulm, Germany
1999	Dr. Evelin F Gevers	Rotterdam, The Netherlands
	Dr. Heiko Krude	Berlin, Germany
2000	Dr. Jörg Dötsch	Erlangen, Germany
2001	Dr. Ken Ong	Cambridge, UK
2002	Dr. John Achermann	London, UK
	Dr. Annemie Boehmer	Rotterdam, The Netherlands
2003	Dr. Delphine Jaquet	Paris, France
	Dr. José Morenos	Amsterdam, The Netherlands
2004	Dr. Taneli Raivio	Helsinki, Finland
2005	Dr. Christa Flück	Berne, Switzerland
2006	Dr. Mirelle Castanet	Paris, France
2007	Dr. Antje Körner	Leipzig, Germany
2008	Dr. Luisa de Sanctis	Turin, Italy
2009	Dr. Felix Riepe	Kiel, Germany
2010	Dr. Martine Cools	Ghent, Belgium
2011	Dr. Helen Storr	London, UK
	Dr. Nils Krone	Birmingham, UK

Outstanding Clinician Award

The Outstanding Clinician Award was established in 2001 with the sponsorship of Pharmacia, Stockholm (now Pfizer) and recognises outstanding clinical contribution to the practice of Clinical Paediatric Endocrinology. The award is open to all ESPE members. without any age limitation. It is given on the basis of nominations received from ESPE members and the winner is selected by the Andrea Prader Prize committee.

Previous Winners		
2001	Dr. Dagfinn Aarskog	Bergen, Norway
2002	Dr. Jaakko Perheentupa	Helsinki, Finland
2003	Dr. Otto Westphal	Gothenburg, Sweden

Previous Winners		
2004	Dr. Emanuele Cacciari	Bologna, Italy
2005	Dr. Jean-Claude Job	Paris, France
2006	Dr. Ruth Illig	Zurich, Switzerland
2007	Dr. Catherine Dacou-Voutetakis	Athens, Greece
2008	Dr. Ferenc Péter	Budapest, Hungary
2009	Dr. Giuseppe Chiumello	Milan, Italy
2010	Dr. Herwig Frisch	Vienna, Austria
2011	Dr. Isis Ghali	Cairo, Egypt

ESPE Research Fellowship

This Fellowship succeeded the Nordisk Grant for the Study of the Growth, which was established in 1978 on the initiative of Professor Andrea Prader, the late Professor Henning Andersen and the late Henry Brennum (Nordisk Gentofte A/S). The ESPE Research Fellowship, sponsored by Novo Nordisk A/S, Copenhagen, supports and finances young paediatricians or scientists, who are intent on a scientific career in paediatric endocrinology, during their research training for up to 2 years.

Previous Winners		
1991	Dr. Päivi J. Tapanainen	Oulu, Finland
1992	Dr. Christina K. Gantenbein	Athens, Greece
	Dr. Claudine Heinrichs	Brussels, Belgium
	Dr. Luis Perez-Jurado	Madrid, Spain
	Dr. Leo Dunkel	Helsinki, Finland
	Dr. Martin Wabitsch	Ulm, Germany
1993	Dr. Catherine Le Stunff	Paris, France
	Dr. Päivi J. Miettinen	Helsinki, Finland
1994	Dr. Barbara Funk	Giessen, Germany
	Dr. Lars Sävendahl	Stockholm, Sweden
	Dr. Francisco Miralles	Barcelona, Spain
1995	Dr. Nicholas Bishop	Cambridge, UK
	Dr. Alessandra Vottero	Parma, Italy
1996	Dr. Silvia González-Parra	Madrid, Spain
	Dr. Ewa Lichtarowicz-Krynsk	London, UK
1997	Dr. José Carlos Monero	Madrid, Spain
	Dr. Sylvie Tenoutasse	Brussels, Belgium
1998	Dr. Thomas Siebler	Leipzig, Germany
	Dr. Nathalie Alos	Narbonne, France

Previous Winners		
1999	Dr. Beate Doecker	Datteln, Germany
	Dr. Sabine Heger	Kiel, Germany
2000	Dr. Jarmo Jääskeläinen	Kuopio, Finland
	Dr. Joachim Woelfle	Bonn, Germany
2001	Dr. Birgit Köhler	Marburg, Germany
	Dr. Outimaija Makitie	Hyks, Finland
2002	Dr. Svetlana Lajic	Stockholm, Sweden
	Dr. Daniel Iliev	Sofia, Bulgaria
2003	Dr. Agnès Linglart	Paris, France
	Dr. Martine Cools	Antwerp, Belgium
2004	Dr. Kathleen de Waele	Ghent, Belgium
	Dr. Catarina Limbert-Zinterl	Lisbon, Portugal
2005	Dr. Dominika Janus	Krakow, Poland
	Dr. Maria Loredana Marcovecchio	Chieti, Italy
2006	Dr. Kyriaki-Sandy Alatzoglou	London, UK
	Dr. Diane Rottembourg	Paris, France
2007	Dr. Delphine Fradin	Paris, France
	Dr. Stephen O'Riordan	Dublin, Ireland
2008	Dr. John Idkowiak	Dresden, Germany
	Dr. Claire Hughes	Dublin, Ireland
2009	Dr. Lysy Philippe	Brussels, Belgium
	Dr. Pamela Schrumpf	Berlin, Germany
2010	Dr. Yvonne van der Zwan	Rotterdam, The Netherlands
	Dr. Christian M. Moya	Madrid, Spain

ESPE Clinical Fellowship

This Fellowship was established with the support of Ares-Serono SA, Geneva, to promote the development of patient care and clinical research in paediatric endocrinology through a training programme. Encouraged by the opening up of Eastern Europe, it was designed for centres where training in paediatric endocrinology is not adequate in the home situation.

Previous Winners		
1993	Dr. Ingrida Pozarska	Riga, Latvia
1994/95	Dr. Vallo Tillmann	Tartu, Estonia
	Dr. Julia Boiko	Minsk, Belarus

Previous Winners			
1996		Dr. Rodica Cornean	Cluj-Napoca, Romania
1997		Dr. Marina Krstevska-Konstantinova	Skopje, Macedonia
1998		Dr. Ihor Hrytsiuk	Lviv, Ukraine
		Violeta Iotova	Varna, Bulgaria
1999		Dr. Oleg Rimizov	Moscow, Russia
		Dr. Oksana Shably	Kiev, Ukraine
		Dr. Marek Niedziela	Poznan, Poland
		Dr. Daniel Iliev	Sofia, Bulgaria
2000		Dr. Elzbieta Perticzko	Szcecin, Poland
		Dr. Julia Titova	St Petersburg, Russia
2001		Dr. Umaima Salem Aboushof	Tripoli, Libya
		Dr. John Torpiano	Malta
		Dr. Luminita Beldean	Sibiu, Romania
		Dr. Antonela Burlacu	Bucharest, Romania
		Dr. Christina Dumitrescu	Bucharest, Romania
		Dr. Iveta Dzivite	Riga, Lativa
		Dr. Galina Popova	Sofia, Bulgaria
		Dr. Ancuta Tudorancea	Arad, Romania
		Dr. Nicolina Dumitriu	Bucharest, Romania
		Dr. Tatjana Milenkovic	Belgrade, Yugoslavia
		Dr. Ann Nordenström	Stockholm, Sweden
2002		Dr. Nicolina Dimitriu	Bucharest, Romania
		Dr. Enver Simsek	Konuralp-Duzce, Turkey
		Dr. Filiz Cizmecioglu	Istanbul, Turkey
		Dr. Sema Kalkan	Izmir, Turkey
2003		Dr. Zdenek Sumnik	Prague, Czech Republic
		Dr. Adriana Dankovcíková	Kosice, Slovakia
		Dr. Zdenek Sumnik	Prague, Czech Republic
		Dr. Adriana Dankovcíková	Kosice, Slovakia
		Dr. Rasa Verkauskiene	Kaunas, Lithuania
		Dr. Maria Kalina	Katowice, Poland
		Dr. Dominika Janus	Krakow, Poland
2004		Dr. Meropi Toumba	Nicosia, Cyprus
		Dr. Aleksandra Górska	Kraków, Poland
2005		Dr. Sudha Rao Chandrashekhar	Mumbai, India
		Dr. Rafael Mantovani	Belo Horizonte, Brazil
		Dr. Balázs Gellén	Szeged, Hungary
		Dr. Malgorzata Kumorowicz-Kopiec	Krakow, Poland

Previous Winners		
2006	Trapaidze Tamari	Tbilisi, Georgia
	Waqas Imran Khan	Multan, Pakistan
	Edna Siima Majaliwa	Muhimbili, Tanzania
	Natalja Kulakova	Tartu, Estonia
	Thomas Ngwiri	Embu, Kenya
	Adriana Beletato dos Santos Balancieri	Florianopolis, Brazil
2007	Veselin Boyadzhiev	Varna, Bulgaria
	David Neumann	Czech Republic
	Hradec Kralove	Czech Republic
	Maria Ionela Pascanu	Tg. Mures, Romania
	Charilaos Stylianou	Thessaloniki, Greece
	Karina De Ferran	Rio de Janeiro, Brazil
	Hasan Abdel Malek Eideh	East Jerusalem, Palestinian Authority
	Falucar Njuieyon	Yaounde, Cameroon
2008	Natalija Tkacenko	Kaunas, Lithuania
	Rita Bertalan	Veszprém, Hungary
	Hinde Iraqi	Rabat, Morocco
	Leila Essaddam	Tunis, Tunisia
	Su Zhe	Guangzhou, PR China
	Elham Mohammad Al Amiri	Sharjah, UAE
	Rajesh Ravindra Joshi	Mumbai, India
	Riatto Della Coletta	Sao Paulo, Brazil
2009	Mary Slessor Limbe	Nairobi, Kenya
	Elena Novikova	Moscow, Russia
	Svetlana Soboleva	Orenburg, Russia
	Hanna Huopio	Kuopio, Finland
	Shakhrizada Sultanova	Tashkent, Uzbekistan
	Tetyana Chaychenko	Kharkiv, Ukraine
	Basim Al-Zoubi	Amman, Jordan
	Asma Ahmed	Karachi, Pakistan
	Lara Vieira Marcal	Belo Horizonte-Minas Gerais, Brazil
	Yuan Xiao	Shanghai, PR China
	Abtisam Mis Tahar Ahdid	Tripoli, Libya
	Paul Laigong	Nairobi, Kenya
	Sofia Leka	Athens, Greece
	Ruiz-Arana Inge Lore	Madrid, Spain
	Giannini Cosimo	Chieti, Italy

Previous Winners		
2010	Cristina Bejnariu	Brasov, Romania
	Simonida Spasevska	Skopje, Macedonia
	Hanane Latrech	Rabat, Morocco
	Iroro Yarhere	Port Harcourt, Nigeria
	Nezha Iraqi	Rabat, Morocco
	Andrea Bischof-Renner	Basel, Switzerland
	Juliana van de Sande Lee	Florianopolis, Brazil
	Safia Zoubir	Oran, Algeria
	Ahmed Ayadi	Sfax, Tunisia
	Vilhelm Mladenov	Varna, Bulgaria
	Imane Benabbad	Rabat, Morocco

ESPE Sabbatical Leave Programme

This programme was established with the support of Eli-Lilly International Corp., London, to enable ESPE members to take a sabbatical leave in order to undertake research in another institution, thereby providing a unique opportunity for scientific renewal, new research development an the establishment of collaborative links.

Previous Winners		Host
1993	David Milner (died 1996)	Sheffield, England
	Tomasz Romer	Warsaw, Poland
1994	Michael Preece	London, England
1995	Not awarded	
1996	Alex Eberle	Basel, Switzerland
	Marc Maes	Brussels, Belgium
	Raimo Voutilainen	Kuopio, Finland
1997	Not awarded	
1998	Cecilia Camacho-Hübner	London, England
1999	Marie-Christine Lebrethon	Liège, Belgium

Previous Winners			Host
2000	Chris Kelnar	Edinburgh, Scotland	
	Ursula Kuhnle-Krahl	Munich, Germany	
2001	Ursula Kuhnle-Krahl	Munich, Germany	
	Jeremy Wales	Sheffield, England	
	Niels Birkebaek	Aarhus, Denmark	
	Heike Jung	Hanover, Germany	
	Nurgun Kandemir	Ankara, Turkey	
2002	Jeremy Wales	Sheffield, England	
2003	Serge Lumbroso	Nimes, France	
	Christian Roth	Bonn, Germany	
2004	Pal Njolstad	Bergen, Norway	Ronald Kahn, USA
	Christian Roth	Bonn, Germany	Sergio Ojeda, USA
2005	Ieuan Hughes	Cambridge, UK	Joseph Majzoub, USA and Peter Gluckman, New Zealand
	Irène Netchine	Paris, France	Pinchas Cohen, USA
2006	Jan Maarten Wit	Leiden, Netherlands	Michael Ranke, Germany
2007	Primus Mullis: Rescuing autosomal-dominant growth hormone deficiency type II	Bern, Switzerland	Iain Robinson, UK
	Jacques Pantel: The ghrelin system in the zebra fish model	Paris, France	R.D. Cone, USA

Previous Winners			Host
2008	Ze'ev Hochberg	Haifa, Israel	Peter Gluckman, New Zealand
	Theo Sas: The role of plasma protein-A in pre- and postnatal growth	Ridderkerk, The Netherlands	Yves Le Bouc, France
2009	Wieland Kiess	Leipzig, Germany	George Werther, Australia
	Fabrizio Barbetti: RNA-based therapy for infancy onset diabetes caused by mutations of the insulin gene	Rome, Italy	Domenico Accili, New York, USA
2010	Serap Turan: The temporal profile of Gs imprinting and XLs expression in the renal proximal tubule during the early postnatal period in mice	Istanbul, Turkey	Henry Kronenberg and Murat Bastepe, Boston, USA
	Jorma Toppari: Importance of normal testicular development for male reproductive health	Turku, Finland	Anders Juul, Copenhagen, Denmark

ESPE Visiting Scholarship

This programme was initiated in 1993 and enables members of the Society to gather information and experience on a specific research problem or on a laboratory technique in the field of paediatric endocrinology. Up to ten scholarships can be awarded each year and cover expenses for a short visit to a different institute. This award is made possible by the generous support of Pharmacia, Sweden, now Pfizer, USA.

Henning Andersen Prize

This prize, which was first awarded in 1986, is given to the best abstract after blind rating, accepted at the Annual Scientific Meeting of the Society. From 1995 two awards are made annually for the most highly rated clinical (c) and experimental (e) abstracts. The prize is sponsored by Novo-Nordisk A/S, Copenhagen, Denmark, in memory of Professor Henning Andersen, one of the founding fathers of ESPE.

Previous Winners		
1986	Dr. Marc Maes	Brussels, Belgium
1987	Dr. Sylvie Hardouin	Paris, France
1988	Dr. Gila Maor	Haifa, Israel
1989	Dr. Raimo Voutilainen	Kuopio, Finland
1990	Dr. Jesús Argente	Madrid, Spain
1991	Dr. Gérald Theintz	Lausanne, Switzerland
1992	Dr. Jean-Pierre Bourguignon	Liège, Belgium
1993	Dr. Walter Miller	San Francisco, USA
1994	Dr. Jean-Pierre Bourguignon	Liège, Belgium
1995	Dr. Angela Weber (c)	London, UK
	Dr. Jean-Marc Lobaccaro (e)	Montpellier, France
1996	Dr. Ze'ev Hochberg (c)	Haifa, Israel
	Dr. Jean-Marc Lobaccaro (e)	Aubiere, France
1997	Dr. James Freeth (c)	Manchester, UK
	Dr. Tamar Amit (e)	Haifa, Israel
1998	Dr. Hanna Huopio (c)	Kuopio, Finland
	Dr. Mehul Dattani (e)	London, UK
1999	Dr. Lourdes Ibanez (c)	Barcelona, Spain
	Dr. Karen Cosgrove (e)	Sheffield, UK
2000	Dr. Julian Hamilton Shield (c)	Bristol, UK
	Dr. A. Vottero (e)	Israel
2001	Dr. Rebecca Perry (c)	Montreal, Canada
	Dr. Anne-Marie Pulichino (e)	Montreal, Canada
2002	Dr. Angela Hübner (c)	Dresden, Germany
	Dr. Sabine Heger (e)	Leipzig, Germany
2003	Dr. Timo Otonkoski (c)	Helsinki, Finland
	Dr. José C. Moreno (e)	Amsterdam, The Netherlands
2004	Dr. Delphine Jaquet/Dr. Julia Boiko (c)	Paris, France/Minsk, Belarus
	Dr. Christian Roth (e)	Bonn, Germany
2005	Dr. Daniele Di Marzio (c)	Chieti, Italy
	Dr. Christina E Hoei-Hansen (e)	Copenhagen, Denmark
2006	Dr. Irène Netchine (c)	Paris, France
	Dr. Ken McElreavey (e)	Paris, France
2007	Dr. Birgit Kohler (c)	Berlin, Germany
	Dr. Evangelia Charmandari (e)	Leeds, UK
2008	Dr. Klaus Mohnike (c)	Magdeburg, Germany
	Dr. Remco Visser (e)	Leiden, Netherlands

Previous Winners		
2009	Dr. Maria Lundgren (c)	Uppsala, Sweden
	Dr. Chloe Pass (e)	Midlothian, UK
2010	Dr. Michael P. Whyte (c)	St. Louis, USA
	Dr. Carles Gaston-Massuet (e)	London, UK

Travel Grants

Travel grants are available for attendance of the annual congress if the applicant has submitted a high quality abstract.

ESPE-Hormone Research in Paediatrics Prize

The annual *ESPE-Hormone Research in Paediatrics prize*, initiated in 2004, rewards a young clinical or experimental scientist for the 'best original paper' published in *Hormone Research in Paediatrics*. The Editor in Chief and the Associate Editors of *Hormone Research in Paediatrics* make up the Selection Committee and potential winners are elected in the spring. The decision is notified to the authors by July. The prize is generously offered by the journal's publisher S. Karger. It is awarded at the ESPE Annual meeting and given to the first author of the winning article.

Previous Winners	
2004	Tenoutasse S, Van Vliet G, Ledru E, Deal C: IGF-I transcript levels in whole-liver tissue, in freshly isolated hepatocytes, and in cultured hepatocytes from lean and obese Zucker rats. Horm Res 2003;59:135–141
2005	de Boer L, Kant SG, Karperien M, van Beers L, Tjon J, Vink GR, van Tol D, Dauwerse H, le Cessie S, Beemer FA, van der Burgt I, Hamel BCJ, Hennekam RC, Kuhnle U, Mathijssen IB, Veenstra-Knol HE, Schrander Stumpel CT, Breuning MH, Wit JM: Genotype-phenotype correlation in patients suspected of having Sotos syndrome. Horm Res 2004;62:197–207
2006	Holterhus PM, Salzburg J, Werner R, Hiort O: Transactivation properties of wild-type and mutant androgen receptors in transiently transfected primary human fibroblasts. Horm Res 2005;63:152–158

Previous Winners	
2007	Best 'Original Paper': Salgin B, Amin R, Yuen K, Williams RM, Murgatroyd P, Dunger DB: Insulin resistance is an intrinsic defect independent of fat mass in women with Turner's syndrome. Horm Res 2006; 65:69–75 Best 'Novel Insights from Clinical Practice': Ostermann S, Salvi R, Lang-Muritano M, Voirol M-J, Puttinger R, Gaillard RC, Schoenle E, Pralong FP: Importance of genetic diagnosis of DAX-1 deficiency: example from a large, multigenerational family. Horm Res 2006;65:163–168
2008	Best 'Original Paper': Hoogendam J, Farih-Sips H, van Beek E, Löwik CWGM, Wit JM, Karperien M: Novel late response genes of PTHrP in Chondrocytes. Horm Res 2007;67:159–170 Best 'Novel Insights from Clinical Practice': Herzovich V, Vaiani E, Marino R, Dratler G, Lazzati JM, Tilitzky S, Ramirez P, Iorcansky S, Rivarola MA, Belgorosky A: Unexpected peripheral markers of thyroid function in a patient with a novel mutation of the MCT8 thyroid hormone transporter gene. Horm Res 2007;67:1–6
2009	Best 'Original Paper': Mallet E, Working Group on Calcium Metabolism: Primary Hyperparathyroidism in Neonates and Childhood. Horm Res 2008;69:180–188 Best 'Novel Insights from Clinical Practice': Mohnike K, Blankenstein O, Pfuetzner A, Pötzsch S, Schober E, Steiner S, Hardy OT, Grimberg A, van Waarde WM: Long-term non-surgical therapy of severe persistent congenital hyperinsulinism with glucagon. Horm Res 2008;70:59–64
2010	Best 'Original Paper': Eldar-Geva T, Hirsch HJ, Rabinowitz R, Benarroch F, Rubinstein O, Gross-Tsur V: Primary ovarian dysfunction contributes to the hypogonadism in women with Prader-Willi syndrome. Horm Res 2009;72:153–159 Best 'Novel Insights from Clinical Practice': Starzyk J, Wójcik M, Wojtyś J, Tomasik P, Mitkowska Z, Pietrzyk JJ: Ovarian hyperstimulation syndrome in newborns – a case presentation and literature review. Horm Res 2009;71:60–64
2011	Best 'Original Paper': Lee S-J, Lee S-H, Ha N-C, Park B-J: Estrogen prevents senescence through induction of WRN, Werner syndrome protein. Horm Res Paediatr 2010;74:33–40 Best 'Novel Insights from Clinical Practice': Kumaran A, Kapoor RR, Flanagan SE, Ellard S, Hussain K: Congenital hyperinsulinism due to a compound heterozygous *ABCC8* mutation with spontaneous resolution at eight weeks. Horm Res Paediatr 2010;73:287–292

ESPE President Poster Awards

The ESPE President Poster Awards are awarded to the five best posters on display at the annual meeting and were first awarded at the 2007 ESPE Annual Meeting in Helsinki. The ESPE President Poster Awards are bestowed by the Programme Organizing Committee members to the presenting and first author of the five selected posters. The selection criteria are based on the scientific content and on the quality of the poster presentation. The five awarded posters are selected from the 50 poster abstracts which attained the best ratings during the abstract evaluation process.

The winners are announced by the President of the meeting during the ESPE President Poster Awards session held prior to the closing ceremony. Each award consists of an official ESPE award diploma, a presidential gift and a citation in the list of ESPE award winners.

Further details are available at http://www.eurospe.org/awards/awards_President Poster.html.

Index to pp. 1–125

Aim, ESPE 7
Åkerblom, Hans 125
Albertsson-Wikland, Kerstin 74, 109
Anand, Kanwal 116
Andersen, Henning 4, 7, 8, 14, 26, 29, 119, 120
Andrea Prader Prize 28, 29, 76, 90, 99, 109, 125
Annual Business Meeting, ESPE 50–52, 108, 109
Annual Meeting concerts 81, 82
Annual Meetings, ESPE 9, 10, 14, 15, 41, 42, 45
Antonin, Francés 83
Argente, Jesús 63, 64, 113
Aubert, Michel 25
Avbelj, Magdalena 92
Aynsley-Green, Al 24, 25, 33, 34, 38, 88, 116

Bartsocas, Christos 91
Battelino, Tadej 92
Belgian Study Group for Paediatric Endocrinology 65–67
Belgium perspective 65–67
Bergstrand, Carl-Gustav 4, 7, 14, 24, 107
Bertrand, Jean 7
Bidlingmaier, Frank 115
Bierich, Jürgen 4, 7, 8, 10, 24, 115
Blizzard, Bob 75
Bluetooth, Harald 120
Blum, Wever 86
Blunck, Werner 116
Bourguignon, Jean-Pierre 65–67, 91
Brennum, Henry 29
Brook, Charles 88, 100, 123
Butenandt, Otfrid 115
Büyükgebiz, Atilla 54

Camacho-Hübner, Cecilia 56
Cathro, Methven 7
Chatelain, Pierre 91
Chiarelli, Francesco 54, 55, 114, 124, 125
Chiumello, Giuseppe 71, 72
Clinical Fellowship, ESPE 35, 97
Clinical Practice Committee, ESPE 47, 49
Confederation of European Societies in Paediatrics 39
Congenital adrenal hyperplasia 6, 14, 78, 91, 96
Congrex Stockholm, ESPE utilization 43–45
Constitution, ESPE 7, 8, 15, 16, 52, 114
Coordination Office of Pediatric Endocrine Societies 32
Corbeel, Lucien 4
Corporate Liaison Board, ESPE 46, 114
Craen, Rita 65, 66
Crowley, W.F. 93
Czechoslovakia perspective 96–99
Czernichow, Paul 23, 25, 26, 73–75, 91, 92, 102, 108

Dacou-Voutetakis, Catherine 76–78, 85
Darendeliler, Feyza 79, 80
Delange, Francois 96
Delemarre-van der Waal, Henriette 97
Denmark perspective 119–121
DiGeorge, A.M. 77
Donaldson, Malcolm 86, 98
Drop, Stenvert 37, 81, 82, 111
Drugs and Therapeutics Committee 39
Du Caju, Marc 65, 66
Dumic, Miro 104
Dunkel, Leo 64, 125

Education and Training Committee, ESPE 47–49

Ernould, Christian 65, 66
Ethics, ESPE screening of abstracts 29–31, 36
European Board of Paediatrics 39
European Society of Endocrinology 35
European Thyroid Association 19

Fanconi, Guido 14
Fanconi Jr., Andreas 4, 7, 24
Ferrier, Pierre 4, 24
Finance Committee, ESPE 47
Finland perspective 122–125
Fisher, Delbert 86
Forest, Maguelone 96
François, René 4, 7, 8, 24, 71
Francés Antonin, José M. 4, 7, 14
Frisch, Herwig 91, 97, 99

Gardner, Lytt 13
Gautier, Emile 4, 7
Global Paediatric Endocrinology and Diabetes 58, 78
González-Parra, Silvia 64
Greece perspective 103
Greenwood, Lorraine 112
Gregory, John 56
Growth hormone therapy 30, 31, 39, 66, 96
Grueters-Kieslich, Annette 85–87
Grumbach, Mel 88, 90
Gunnarsson, Rolf 97

Habich, Hans 4
Hagedorn, H.C. 119
Hamilton, William 7, 8, 11, 71
Hamza, Rasha 98
Helge, Hans 34, 85, 115
Henning Andersen Prize 26, 28, 63, 124, 125
Hesse, Volker 34, 89
Hnikova, Olga 96
Hochberg, Ze'ev 36, 53, 76, 78, 86, 89, 91, 97, 99, 108, 109, 125
Hormone Research 32, 34, 48, 56
Hormone Research in Paediatrics 48
Hormone Research in Paediatrics Prize 59
Hubble, Douglas 4, 7, 10, 13
Hübner, Angela 98
Hughes, Leuan 21, 29, 74, 88–90
Huix, F.J. 4
Huopio, Hanna 125

Illig, Ruth 4, 7, 14, 24, 63, 71, 83, 91, 96, 123
International Study Group on Diabetes in Children and Adolescents 91, 95
Iodine deficiency 96
Iotova, Violeta 97

Jääskeläinen, Jarmo 125
Job, Jean-Claude 15, 30, 63
Jost, Alfred 74
Juul, Anders 64

Kaplan, Selna 75, 123
Kastrup, Knud W. 119–121
Kelnar, Chris 97
Key Committee, ESPE 47
Kiess, Wieland 64, 86
Knip, Mikael 125
Knorr, Dieter 4, 7, 15, 21, 22, 24, 115
Knorr-Mürset, Gertrud 4, 7, 14, 22, 24, 83
Kolousková, Stanislava 96
Korth-Schütz, Sigrun 85
Kotnok, Primoz 92
Krzisnik, Ciril 91–93, 97

Laron, Zvi 4, 7, 10, 12, 24, 63, 71, 89, 91, 94, 95, 100, 124
Lawson Wilkins Pediatric Endocrine Society, ESPE joint meetings 20, 32, 89, 94, 95, 102, 106, 108, 113, 124
Lebl, Jan 91, 96–99
Leger, Juliane 86
Lestradet, Henry 91, 95
Loeb, Helmuth 95
Longás, Angel Ferrández 83

Maes, Marc 56, 65–67, 125
Maghreb Project, ESPE 57
Majaliwa, Edna 98
Mäkitie, Outi 125
Malvaux, Paul 7, 65–67
Mantovani, Rafael 97
Maor, Gila 28
Matajac, Leo 91
Matsaniotis, N. 77
Membership, ESPE
  Eastern Bloc countries 37
  growth 16, 37, 53
  requirements 9, 17
Memorial Forest, ERSPE 55
Miettinen, Päivi 124, 125
Migeon, Claude J. 20

Miller, Walter 122–124
Misokiva, Zelmira 91
Money, John 15
Moreno, José Carlos 64
Mullis, Primus 100–102
Mürset, Gertrud, *see* Knorr-Mürset, Gertrud

Nairobi Training Centre 56, 99
New Inroads in Child Health 60
New, Maria 13, 77, 85, 103, 104
Newsletter, ESPE 48, 64
Neyzi, Olcay 80, 91
Nielsen, Jakob 92
Nilsson, Lars R. 4, 7

Okolo, Angela 56
Otonkoski, Timo 124, 125
Outstanding Clinician Award, ESPE 40, 99

Paediatric and Adolescent Gynaecology Working Group 67
Paediatric Endocrine Society 94
Paediatric Endocrinology in Developing Countries 56
Paulsen, Frederik 74, 75, 90
Pérez-Jurado, Luis 64
Perheentupa, Jaakko 122
Péter, Ferenc 34, 91, 116
Pierson, Michel 7, 10
Polak, Michel 64
Poster sessions, ESPE 18, 58
Prader, Andrea 3, 4, 6–10, 13, 14, 24, 28, 29, 63, 71, 76, 77, 83, 85, 95, 101
Prader-Willi syndrome 92
President's Poster Award, ESPE 59
Programme Organising Committee 38, 39, 41–44, 46, 47, 59, 105, 106

Raiti, Salvatore 20
Raivio, Taneli 125
Ranke, Michael 96, 102, 116
Rao, Sudha 98
Rappaport, Raphaël 7, 19, 38, 41, 71, 105, 106
Razzaghy-Azar, Maryam 51, 112, 113
Recent Progress in Paediatric Endocrinology 60
Research Award, ESPE 40, 109, 125
Research Fellowship, ESPE 29
Ritzén, Martin 44, 56, 74, 91, 92, 107–110
Rochiccioli, Pierre 75

Romer, Tomasz 37
Rossi, Ettore 13, 76
Royer, Pierre 7, 73, 105

Sabbatical Leave Programme, ESPE 39, 125
Saenger, Paul 54
Savage, Martin 46, 50, 111–114, 124
Scarf, ESPE 33
Schärer, Karl 4
Schoenle, Eugen 95
Schönberg, Dieter 115
Schwenk, Alfred 4, 7, 24
Science School, ESPE 60
Shalet, Steven 42, 46, 102, 113
Sippell, Wolfgang 91, 115–118, 124
Sizonenko, Pierre 17, 20, 21, 44, 74, 81, 102
Skakkebaek, Niels 28, 89, 119–121
Slovenia perspective 91–93
Sobel, Edna 13
Söder, Olle 86
Spahr, André 4
Spain perspective 83, 84
Stalder, Gerhard 4
Steendjik, Robert 4, 7, 24
Strategic Planning Committee 46
Sultan, Charles 97
Summer School, ESPE 25–27, 73, 74, 80, 86, 91, 92, 108
Sweden perspective 105–110
Switzerland perspective 100–102
Swoboda, Walter 7, 13, 15

Tanner, James M. 7, 77
Tansek, Mojca 92
Tapanainen, Juha 123
Tapanainen, Päivi 123, 125
Teller, Walter 7, 19, 115
Thamdrup, Erik 120
Tie, ESPE 33
Tjulpalov, Anatolij 97
Turner Syndrome Working Group 78

Van den Brande, Leo 43, 51, 74, 97, 101
van der Werff ten Bosch, Koos 7
Vandeweghe, Marc 65, 66
Van Vliet, Guy 65, 66
Van Wyk, Judson 13, 107
Verkauskiene, Rasa 97
Vest, Markus 4, 7, 24
Villee, Claude 10
Villee, Dorothy 10

Visiting Scholarship, ESPE 36
Visser, Henk 4–8, 9, 10, 11, 13, 15, 18, 20, 24, 77, 81, 117
Voerste, Joanna 117
Voutilainen, Ralmo 122–125

Weber, Bruno 34
Werner, Egon 4, 7
Westphal, Otto 56
Wilkins, Lawson 6, 20, 107, 119, 120
Winter, Jeremy 88

Winter School, ESPE 35, 36, 80, 92, 97, 98, 109
Wolter, Renée 65, 66
World Diabetes Foundation 56

Yearbook of Paediatric Endocrinology 48
Young Investigator Award, ESPE 40

Zachmann, Milo 14, 15, 17, 20, 28, 29, 63, 77, 83, 102, 105
Zuppinger, Klaus 100